MW00528526

STARVING TO HEAL IN SIBERIA

MY RADICAL RECOVERY FROM LATE-STAGE LYME DISEASE AND HOW IT COULD HELP OTHERS

STARVING TO HEAL IN SIBERIA

MICHELLE B. SLATER, PH.D.

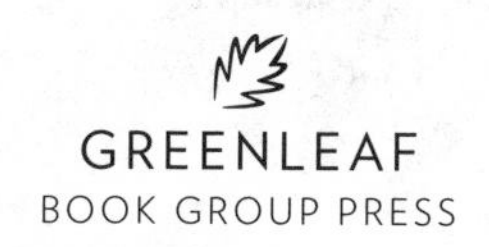

GREENLEAF
BOOK GROUP PRESS

This book is intended as a reference volume only, not as a medical manual. The information given here is designed to help you make informed decisions about your health. It is not intended as a substitute for any treatment that may have been prescribed by your doctor. If you suspect that you have a medical problem, you should seek competent medical help. You should not begin a new health regimen without first consulting a medical professional.

Published by Greenleaf Book Group Press
Austin, Texas
www.gbgpress.com

Copyright © 2022 Michelle B. Slater

All rights reserved.

Thank you for purchasing an authorized edition of this book and for complying with copyright law. No part of this book may be reproduced, stored in a retrieval system, or transmitted by any means, electronic, mechanical, photocopying, recording, or otherwise, without written permission from the copyright holder.

Distributed by Greenleaf Book Group

For ordering information or special discounts for bulk purchases, please contact Greenleaf Book Group at PO Box 91869, Austin, TX 78709, 512.891.6100.

Design and composition by Greenleaf Book Group
Cover design by Greenleaf Book Group
Cover Image: ©Shutterstock/Vitalii Matokha

Grateful acknowledgment is made to the following for permission to reproduce copyrighted material:

Counterpoint Press and Wendell Berry: Excerpt from "The Reassurer" from *New Collected Poems*. Copyright © 1994 by Wendell Berry. Reprinted with the permission of The Permissions Company, LLC on behalf of Counterpoint Press, counterpointpress.com.
Danna Faulds: From "Allow," in *Go In and In: Poems from the Heart of Yoga* by Danna Faulds. Copyright © 2002 by Danna Faulds. All rights reserved.
Liveright/W. W. Norton & Company, Inc.: From "i thank You God for most this amazing," in *Complete Poems, 1904–1962* by E. E. Cummings. Copyright © 1997 by E. E. Cummings. All rights reserved.
W. W. Norton & Company, Inc.: From "How to Be," in *Sun in Days: Poems* by Meghan O'Rourke. Copyright © 2017 by Meghan O'Rourke. All rights reserved.

Publisher's Cataloging-in-Publication data is available.

Print ISBN: 978-1-62634-986-5

eBook ISBN: 978-1-62634-987-2

Part of the Tree Neutral® program, which offsets the number of trees consumed in the production and printing of this book by taking proactive steps, such as planting trees in direct proportion to the number of trees used: www.treeneutral.com

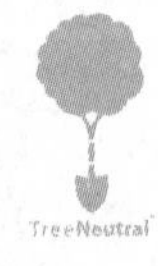

Printed in the United States of America on acid-free paper

22 23 24 25 26 27 28 29 10 9 8 7 6 5 4 3 2 1

First Edition

To my doctor, Sergei Ivanovich, who harnesses the inherent healing capabilities in the human body, and to my "Siberia! Sweet Siberia!" team—Dad, Janet, and Dmitri—for supporting me through this harrowing journey to heal

CONTENTS

FOREWORD

I am grateful to fate that I met an American girl named Michelle who had serious health problems. She had advanced Lyme disease, which triggered an autoimmune disorder, and at the time, she also suffered from candidiasis and psoriasis. She ate a healthy diet; however, she took countless antibiotics that negatively affected her health. Michelle became my patient remotely in July 2017, and she came to us in Siberia that August and stayed with us until October. She conducted several long dry fasts under our care, and she followed my protocol precisely with tremendous results.

Michelle arrived at my clinic with terrible symptoms. She had been bedridden intermittently for several months and could not walk. She had debilitating pain in the joints of her arms and legs, and because of this, she could not sleep at night. She also had constant chronic fatigue from her illness, as well as brain fog and headaches, so she could not think clearly.

I doubted very much that such a thin girl from America would be able to go through such a hard dry fast, but fortunately, I was wrong. She had great motivation and a great desire to recover. But her ability to meditate was the main thing that helped her go through dry fasting as comfortably and efficiently as possible. In my new book on dry fasting, I have included information on the importance of meditation as a foundation for undergoing dry fasting, thanks to witnessing Michelle's experience. I still admire Michelle for her will and her patience, and she is one of the best patients in my practice.

Michelle was one of the first patients to come to me with Lyme disease. After her successful treatment, when she started writing a blog, many Lyme patients came to me in Russia. Michelle's full recovery gave impetus and information to other people who were suffering. Many of the patients who came to me following Michelle were in a severe stage of Lyme disease. Some of them underwent several dry fasting courses (from seven to eleven days), experienced full recoveries, and returned to their former professional and personal activities.

Why did dry fasting help these patients?

The answer is that inflammation cannot exist without water. Any inflamed area of the body swells with water. Only in a moist environment can microbes and viruses multiply. Water deficiency is detrimental to inflammation or any kind of pathological fluid (edema). When the body is dehydrated, a strong competition for water between body cells and pathogens begins. Body cells take water from microorganisms, as well as from the air, absorbing it through the skin. Healthy, strong cells receive additional energy and water, while diseased cells, viruses, and bacteria cannot do this.

Dry fasting also suppresses inflammation through the action of glucocorticoid hormones, which are the body's most powerful anti-inflammatory agent. Glucocorticoid hormones and sex hormones are 70 percent bound by blood transport albumins, and only 30 percent circulate in the blood in a free state. During dry fasting, transport albumins break down, and their amino acids go to the needs of the body—primarily to the needs of the brain and the cardiovascular system. This releases a massive amount of hormones, which circulate in the blood in a free state. At amounts three times more than usual, the glucocorticoids flooding the blood have a strong anti-inflammatory effect, suppressing all the foci of the body's inflammation and resulting in a therapeutic effect in the treatment of autoimmune diseases, such as rheumatoid arthritis.

In addition, during dry fasting, toxins are burned, one might say, in their own furnace; each cell, in the absence of water, triggers an internal thermonuclear reaction. It undergoes an extreme internal process of destruction: everything that is superfluous gets destroyed. Each cell for a while turns into a mini-furnace, a mini-reactor, so there is a powerful cleansing of the body.

The resulting increase in the internal temperature of the body is an important part of the body's protective reactions against disease. At a higher temperature, all metabolic processes in the body are accelerated, so the toxins that cause disease disappear faster, and even cancer cells completely stop their vital activity. It is also known that with an increase in temperature, interferon is more actively released, which gives the body the ability to fight viruses. At high temperatures, antibodies that protect against disease are more actively produced, and phagocytic, bactericidal, and lymphocytic activity increases. All these processes speed up recovery.

Additionally, with the increase in body temperature comes a slowdown in the growth of microorganisms. It becomes easier for the immune system to hunt down and kill everything alien to the body. And without any intake of food or water, the blood does not receive many harmful substances, and it is constantly cleansed by the body. Put simply, the immune system gets a great rest. In this way, dry fasting purifies the blood more perfectly than hemodialysis. As I counsel my patients, if a person prepares by following my medical protocol for dry fasting, then there are practically no complications.

I thank Michelle very much for writing this book, which will help thousands of people achieve full health. I am tremendously grateful to her for sharing her story and the science of dry fasting.

Dr. Sergey Ivanovich Filonov

INTRODUCTION

I'd like to tell you about a place called 1 Bed Avenue. It's where I used to live—sometimes for months at a time. Diagnosed with Lyme disease in 2012, I received outstanding care from the specialists I saw. All the same, I didn't get better. There I was, like so many other people with chronic Lyme and other mystery illnesses—like chronic fatigue or certain autoimmune diseases—that stump doctors. "You'll have to adapt to this new normal," the best of them said, sounding sympathetic, if less than reassuring. My new normal meant taking up residence in my bed—where I spent days that smudged into nights, until, once in a while, I'd have the surreal realization that weeks had passed, much to my chagrin. I did not *choose* to shelter in place confined to a bed. It was untenable; "normal" was its antithesis.

I lived in Connecticut just miles away from the town of Lyme, where the disease was first diagnosed in 1977.[1] Ticks are now ubiquitous in Connecticut and Massachusetts, my stomping grounds for long walks in the woods. I knew to be vigilant in checking for the elusive tiny black vampires after every walk I took, because Lyme disease had become rampant throughout New England (and cases have been reported throughout the United States, Europe, and beyond).

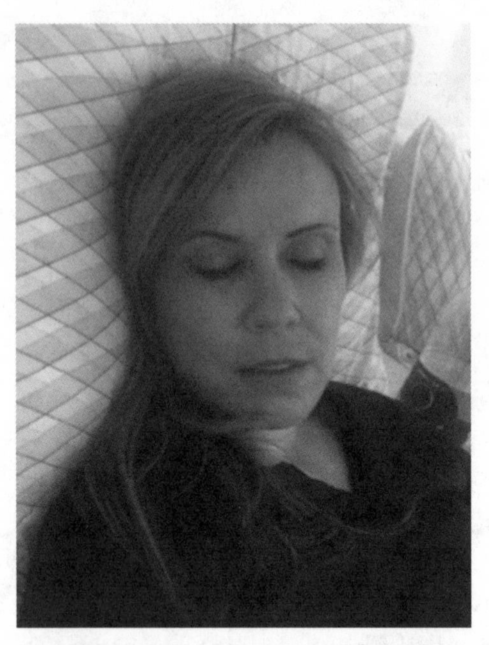

1 Bed Avenue, my place of solace for nearly six years

Lyme, caused by the bacterium *Borrelia burgdorferi* (named after the researcher Willy Burgdorfer, who first identified it), is the most prevalent vector-borne disease in the United States. If one is bitten by a microscopic tick in the genus *Ixodes* that is infected with the bacteria, one has a high likelihood of contracting the disease. Researchers have identified multiple coinfections associated with ticks that transmit *Borrelia burgdorferi*, including *Bartonella*, *Babesia microti*, *Ehrlichia*, and *Anaplasma phagocytophilum*. The *Borrelia* bacterium is a spirochete, one of the most aggressive bacterial forms. Their coiled shape allows them to spiral through the body, employing sophisticated ways of burrowing into the joints, cells, and organs—and even crossing the blood-brain barrier. Because of the miniscule size of the tick, which makes it hard to find once it has burrowed in the body, and the invisible war the spirochetes wage from within, diagnosing Lyme disease is challenging.

Treating Lyme is also problematic. Although it's widely believed that between 70 and 80 percent of infected individuals develop the classic bull's-eye rash known as erythema migrans,[2] I have spoken with countless chronic Lyme patients who, like me, never developed the rash. The common symptoms of fever, migraines, headaches, and fatigue (among multiple others) lead many patients to seek medical attention, but these symptoms can be attributed to numerous other diseases as well. If a patient undergoes laboratory testing and is treated immediately, Lyme disease has a higher chance of being eradicated with antibiotics. But if Lyme disease is undetected and untreated, as mine was, the infection becomes chronic and can spread to the joints, heart, brain, and nervous system. Nearly 10 percent of untreated patients develop neurological problems, or neuroborreliosis, as I did.[3] Mine happened to be one of the unfortunate cases that lapsed into late-stage Lyme disease. Although I had always been careful to check myself for ticks, the tiny vampires had ravaged me, as they have millions of others. Chronic Lyme disease is notoriously challenging to cure.

You may have come to this book because you've been told the same thing I was: that, having exhausted all the options of your caregivers, you should adjust to the "new normal"—which, like me, you may have found devastating. Or you may be a doctor who has had to tell your patients to adjust to the chronic symptoms of an autoimmune disorder or post-treatment Lyme that didn't dissipate under your gold-standard care. Or you may have heard your family members, friends, or colleagues lament the perpetual state of their declining health, as if their former selves had vanished as the insidious disease claimed them—this is a big population of people. Or you may also have read about intermittent fasting and be curious about the research and science behind dry fasting.

What I would like to offer, as the beneficial result of my painful experience, is the antidote to despair for chronically ill patients, as well as for doctors and their circles: there is hope for recovery, and a *complete* recovery, at that. I haven't resided at 1 Bed Avenue for more than an eight-hour stay per night since I discovered that the body could be the doctor. My verve for life came back. Intrigued?

I wrote this narrative just for you, and it takes you from my long-lasting habitat in bed all the way to Siberia, where I was cured through a method called dry fasting. I then delve into the science behind my treatment, and I offer a protocol based on the one that I received from my doctor there, who is the current leader in this method.

I decided to rise up and fight the complex illness plaguing me, and I know I'm not alone in feeling that I could no longer live with being sick but that my disease was mysterious.

Autoimmune disorders are on the rise worldwide, along with "mystery illnesses," such as chronic fatigue syndrome, which elude treatment and recovery. The American Autoimmune Related Diseases Association reports that nearly 50 million Americans have autoimmune disorders,[4] and the National Institutes of Health estimates that 25 million Americans have been diagnosed with an autoimmune disorder.[5]

I believe that the escalation is the signal that it's time to start dry fasting.

Dr. Sergey Filonov, the Siberian doctor who played the pivotal role in my recovery, identifies inflammation as a major contributor to the rise of chronic illnesses and autoimmune disorders. According to recent research, an abnormal inflammatory response is directly related to autoimmune disorders.[6] Additionally, researchers have pinpointed an excess of adipose tissue as a contributor to autoimmune diseases, because adipose tissue creates an inflammatory reaction that activates "adipokines," or pro-inflammatory factors in the body, including leptin, TNF cells, and C-reactive protein.[7] If we have excess adipocytes, then we're activating an immune response that elevates inflammation in the body. Dr. Filonov's protocol for dry fasting, paired with a clean diet that avoids excess fat, sugar, salt, and processed foods, is the greatest weapon against the rise of autoimmune disorders, mystery illnesses such as chronic fatigue, and most notably—in my case—chronic Lyme disease.

As Dr. Filonov explains the efficient process of dry fasting, "Understood as a community of cells, the organism during the fast 'eats' not only the fat cells but also all the elements that are superfluous, morbid or malfunctioning. The continuation of the organism's life is impossible without the self-cleaning of its cell populations. Cells infected with viruses, toxins or damaged by radiation . . . have to either leave the organism or be eaten."[8]

Radical autophagy is the only treatment out of dozens that has cured me, and cure is the right word. One of my doctors in Europe told me during a check-up after I returned from Siberia, "Michelle, if all of my patients went to dry fast in Siberia like you have, I would no longer have a job. That would make me very happy." I have not even had one Lyme symptom since I returned home from Siberia in the fall of 2017; nor have I taken a single pill or supplement of any kind.

I no longer conduct late-night Google searches in desperate search for a cure; nor do I break down sobbing at the state of hopeless decay in my body. Psoriasis, sinus pain, joint pain, migraines, chronic fatigue, brain fog, candida, mold symptoms, insomnia, light sensitivity, and despair are no longer in my life. I no longer have to worry about the nebulous forms of testing for tick-borne diseases that are flawed, for I no longer manifest clinical symptoms. I'm not a scientist, but I know that clearing accumulated waste in my body created a state of health in me that I have not heretofore experienced.

In the chapters that follow, I spell out each step I took and share the embarrassing pitfalls I encountered as I established my healthy routine. In the appendices, I share protocol tips and recipes that contributed to my newfound health. As a person who rarely gives out even my last name, I would only write such a personal memoir if I knew it could help many people; helping you is the reason I have written this book.

PART I

A VERY SICK GIRL

1

VIGNETTES FROM THE LYME TIMELINE

If this last-ditch effort to jumpstart my body did not work, I planned to commit assisted suicide. I don't believe in suicide. I'm a carpe diem, seize-the-day kind of a girl. I wake up in awe of the sunrise, brainstorming what I will do with the gift of a brand-new day. Ever since I read *Walden Pond* as a teenager, I realized that I was always on a quest to suck the marrow out of life. I trekked through the Scottish Highlands from Glasgow to Ben Nevis when I was seventeen and went solo hiking in the Rocky Mountains two years later. I hosted Sunday champagne brunches at Dartmouth that turned into all-nighters, which gave me the nickname "Champagne Miche." In my twenties, I'd stay up late into the night writing my master's theses on Mallarmé poems in French by candlelight. I played classical alto saxophone sonatas and concertos on the Pont des Arts in Paris for fun on Sunday afternoons. I pursued degrees in music performance, literary theory, comparative literature, and French literature until I had a Ph.D. in my hands. I was on my way to becoming a tenured professor, proud to arm my students with critical thinking tools and stoke their creative intellect, when—quite suddenly—the quality of my life deteriorated to the extent that the day had seized me. I wasn't the only one to notice that it had.

The Two Michelles: Dmitri's Account, June 2012

When I dropped Michelle off at John F. Kennedy airport, I rolled my eyes at her insistence on traveling with suitcases full of literary theory books. "Why can't you just put them on a fricking Kindle like a normal person?" I said as I unloaded the hefty cases. Guilt slapped me when I remembered I wouldn't see my wife all summer while she was at her comparative literature summer institute in Istanbul. My scolding didn't seem to faze Michelle, though.

"Oh, but I love these books, and I need to mark up the margins to respond to certain ideas," she said. The excitement in her hazel eyes shone through at me. I looked down at my jeans, scruffy trainers, and half-untucked button-down dress shirt, and then I looked at her styled blond hair and cream linen summer traveling suit. I smiled at her and thought about how divergent our summers would be. I could guarantee that she would not be watching the 2012 Summer Olympics taking place in London.

"The *renowned* literary scholar Erich Auerbach wrote his masterpiece *Mimesis* while exiled in Istanbul, and he didn't even have access to his *library*," she concluded. She had passion, I would give her that, but linen traveling suits and recondite books made her an anachronistic person.

Two months later, I was back at the airport to pick her up. When Michelle limped out into the international arrival hall at JFK, leaning with all her weight against the luggage cart, I realized she hadn't been exaggerating when she told me over the phone that something was drastically wrong.

If she had looked like one of those hot-air balloons soaring over the white alien-like rocks of Cappadocia when she left, that balloon had deflated into near oblivion. She didn't even smile when she saw me. She just blinked her eyes as a greeting and fell into my chest when I went to hug her. I quipped about how glad she must be that all her books made it back safely, but she mumbled that she couldn't read them anymore.

"The words just dance around the page, and I can't make them stay put," she said. Her voice was resigned. There was a heat wave that late August, but she spent the first few days at home bundled in her faded Johns Hopkins sweatshirt under a blanket, eyes closed, shivering. Her beloved dog Brady never left her side, and he barked at me as if he were telling me to fix her. I longed for her to ramble about meeting one of her favorite novelists, Orhan Pamuk. She just slept. Upon waking, she whispered, "The lymph nodes in the roof of my mouth are swollen."

I would offer to put a movie on for her when I left for work, but she said that watching the screen tortured her head and eyes. She mumbled about how she needed to get up and prepare her syllabi, but I wondered how she was going to be able to stand up in front of a classroom when she couldn't seem to remember where the simplest things were in our home. Where had Michelle gone?

Navigating the Maze: From Diagnosis to Treatment

Testing was not proving helpful. I had thought from the outset that I had Lyme disease. I will never forget the day I took a shower in the Berkshires, near the Appalachian Trail in western Massachusetts, and discovered a tiny vampire embedded in my flesh. As I turned to scrub my right shoulder with a soapy washcloth, I saw a black speck wedged in my flesh, wiggling its microscopic legs. Shrieking, I burst out of the shower in search of tweezers, flooding the floor, and scaring Brady, who went into high alert trying to help. I gouged my slippery wet shoulder several times in the wrong places with tweezers until I dug out the remains of the burrowed tick.

This was in 2011. I did everything right. Although I had massacred the tick and my shoulder, I put the mangled tick remains in a plastic bag and took it to the doctor. I got tested. The doctor said I didn't have Lyme.

I muddled on until the symptoms grew strident in the summer of 2012, when I came home from Istanbul. Since I had already tested negative for Lyme, I was most worried about my mind.

During this period, my memory was so unreliable that I left my wedding ring at the massage therapist's office, which she kindly returned to me. I would forget my destination when I was driving, and then I couldn't remember my way home. When I eventually made it there, I would leave my keys in the door. *Was I losing my mind?*

I went to a psychiatrist in Connecticut, seeking an answer. I wasn't alone in going this path. Before the acclaimed author Amy Tan was diagnosed with Lyme disease, she visited a psychiatrist because "something in her had broken."[1]

"Michelle, you are not mentally ill, but I want you to have blood samples taken at the lab," Dr. Tami Amiri reassured me. She called a few days later to announce, "You have Lyme disease!" We laughed about it taking a psychiatrist to diagnose me with Lyme, but the mirth was ephemeral.

After taking the perfunctory dose of 200 mg of doxycycline antibiotics for thirty days, nothing had changed. I felt like I had taken candy instead of medicine. My general practitioner prescribed yet another round for thirty days, but it didn't burn off the fog in my brain; nor did it return my nimble body to me. He told me that it was not advisable to take any more antibiotics, so I gave up for a while.

In the summer of 2014, I launched a nonprofit, the Mayapple Center, a grassroots summer retreat for artists and intellectuals. The work stimulated me, but it drained my reserves. By the end of the summer programming, my symptoms flared up again, until I could only go from my upstairs bedroom to the kitchen by sliding down the stairs on my bottom, one step at a time. The short journey took so much effort that I would lie down on the hardwood floor at the bottom of the stairs and rest for a while. I could no longer drive because I couldn't mold my hands around the steering wheel.

I made an appointment later that summer with a famous Lyme specialist in Connecticut, Dr. Steven Phillips, former president of the International Lyme and Associated Diseases Society. Dr. Phillips was a passionate advocate for going beyond standard prescriptions of antibiotics to heal his patients of Lyme and associated vector-borne diseases, otherwise known in Lyme vernacular as co-infections.

Frustrated by Lyme's tendency to elude standard lab work, Dr. Phillips had become a medical detective. He tested levels of obscure killer cells that I had never heard of, such as CD-57, or immunologic markers that reveal chronic inflammation and autoimmune issues.

"Michelle, your CD-57 levels are at rock bottom," he explained, "which means that your body has been fighting off invaders for a long time." Dr. Phillips told me that, based on my blood work, the Lyme was chronic. It had been with me far earlier than the tick bite I reported in 2011. This didn't shock me, for I had lived with secret symptoms that I worked to conceal for years.

Dr. Phillips's treatment plan involved me taking 1,500 milligram daily doses of tetracycline. Although he explained that the maximum dosage is 2,000 milligrams, it seemed massive to me, since I had taken the standard 200 milligram dose prior to that. He also prescribed 200 milligrams of Diflucan, an antimicrobial medication. My stomach was suffering from the industrial-strength antibiotics, even though he prescribed specially coated pills. When the tick bites a human, it releases spirochetes from its salivary glands into the bloodstream of the host. I persevered through violent reactions as they died off in my body, and I had brief respites from my symptoms, but I didn't recover. We even tried anti-malaria drugs. The gold standard treatment for Lyme is antibiotics, but my body and mind refused to return to me.

I became my own head doctor and went on a quest over the next few years to fight Lyme beyond what allopathic medicine could offer. I tried herbal supplements, functional medicine, heavy metal chelation, Rife machines, mold remediation, homeopathic remedies, Ayurvedic *panchakarma*, far infrared saunas, BioMats, saltwater pools, kinesiology, raw vegan diets, thousands of vitamins and minerals, reiki, deep-tissue massages, acupuncture, Chinese herbs, and a multitude of other treatments in my quest for a cure. None of them helped, and I began to despair.

Jackson Hole, Wyoming, June 2015

And poets are what we need when ill, not prose writers.
In illness words seem to possess a mystic quality.

—Virginia Woolf, *On Being Ill*

I awoke to see the sun rise in shades of periwinkle through the window, filtered through my fog. I wasn't sure where I was, or who I was.

Then I heard Dmitri's familiar voice as he spoke on the phone to someone from work. There was a wedding anniversary card with a photo of a boy holding a rose in his teeth standing on my bedside table. "Ah, Jackson Hole," I sighed. We were here for our fifteenth anniversary, and I had just turned forty.

As the sun rose higher, I felt mocked by the hope of its raspberry rays. There wasn't going to be any horseback riding together through rugged rivers that day, or any vigorous hiking below the spires of the Tetons. Dmitri waved at me from the balcony. The sun caught the golden glint in his hair. Our long-standing code on vacations was that mornings were for working, and we would meet up later; we had always respected one another's work ethics since meeting as students at Dartmouth College. Only I had no work to do.

I pulled on my jeans and sweater and wandered down to the coffee shop on the corner, journal clutched in my aching hands. I sat down with an almond milk latté to scrawl out some words. With each sip and each written word, I tried to find my way out of the fog:

My brain—or is it still a brain—
is floating away in largo tempo,
as if on a lethargic current of air.
Strident calls from my psoas and lumbar
mute my thoughts.
All I hear is their crescendo through my back and limbs,
reminding me that I am in this broken body.

The sun is rising in Jackson Hole
but I am in its shadow
for no raspberry rays shine in these parts.
Where have I to go this morning?

There is no manuscript to write.
There is no class to teach.

Tabula rasa after two master's degrees and a Ph.D.
How does one confront a blank slate, when
one's brain has been replaced with a stranger's brain?
When one's brain is the other?
What can be written on a blank slate when one doesn't
have the
crit-theory brain,
the music brain, the lit brain that one once had?

And this slate? It is broken.
The pieces have been saved,
but they don't fit together.
Shards are missing.
Tabula rasa, on a broken slate,
a failed synecdoche.
Yet.

This discursive narrative
leaves me cleaving to a new handmade
axiom, "One Miche: Lovable As Is"
as if I were a used commodity. As Is.
Crit-theory brain, music brain, lit brain, could not love
this Miche
as is.

Too slow, memory faulty, fallible, unable to produce,
but broken-slate Miche with the other's brain

has had it with these Sisyphean pursuits and echoes
"Lovable As Is."
As is.

Being chronically ill razed my academic drive, my ambitions, and my perfectionism. My lifelong mantra had always been "Strive to achieve." When Lyme vanquished me, it gave me a gift. It took away my fragile sense of self-worth based on what I could accomplish. And, in doing so, it taught me the greatest lesson of my life: I am one Miche, lovable as is. Like one's favorite old station wagon, I am lovable in spite of all my dents and broken bits. I am like the Japanese aesthetic of *wabi sabi*, more beautiful because of my cracks and fissures.

Interlochen, March 2017: The Poster Child for Lyme Disease and Climate Change

Climate change increases the number and geographic range of disease-carrying insects and ticks.

—Centers for Disease Control and Prevention,
"Insects and Ticks"

I would be guest teaching at Interlochen Arts Academy in just one week, but as each late February morning brought me closer to my flight to Traverse City, Michigan, I woke up vacillating between feeling angst and feeling honored. I'd attended Interlochen in high school, and it had formed me. The school sits in the northern Michigan woods, between two lakes, and my time there had stayed in my memory as a sort of educational utopia. There I'd attended Yo-Yo Ma recitals, taken master classes with Branford Marsalis, and majored in music performance. Now, at the request of Professor Mary Ellen Newport, I'd be returning to teach a seminar on ecology and the arts.

It had been three years since I'd taught in a classroom—I'd simply been too sick. But I couldn't refuse the chance to be at Interlochen. Even if it meant that I would have to read and reread and take copious lecture notes because I couldn't trust my memory. I would never let on that I couldn't work more than a few minutes a day at the computer because of migraines and aching fingers that refused to flutter over the keyboard like they once did.

When the time to depart came, I had somehow pieced together a PowerPoint presentation, complete with notes and discussion questions. *Perhaps they won't know how fiercely I had grappled with this?* I could only hope to appear normal.

When I stood before my bright students—all thirty of them—I knew exactly what to say: "You are living in an extraordinary time in the history of this planet. As climatologist Dr. Joseph Romm writes, 'Climate change will have a bigger impact on us and on our families than the internet has.'[2] Can you imagine that?"

My students had just completed a unit on the science of climate change, but they shook their heads. Hal, a dance major, raised his hand and said, "We get the science of it, Dr. Slater. I want to work on representing rising sea levels in my choreography."

I paused to give him some encouragement and continued. "Many of us have been able to displace the idea of climate change, for we have not yet faced crises in our own lives. Our pet polar bears have not died, and the Arctic is a faraway land. Yet how long can climate change remain far, far away?"

Then I shifted it to the personal. "I want you to share with me how—and if—climate change has affected you thus far. I'll go first. I fell prey to an aggressive case of Lyme disease that was diagnosed in 2012. The CDC—the Centers for Disease Control—calls Lyme the first disease directly caused by global warming. Although only 30,000 cases are reported annually, estimates calculate that over 400,000 individuals contract Lyme each year.[3] Do you know anyone with Lyme?" I asked.

Many hands shot up. I could see that my students were looking at me in a new light, as if I were part of the inherent structure of the lesson plan, as if I were right in the messy exhibit of climate change.

It's one thing to stand up in a classroom and label yourself a product of climate change, and it's quite another thing to live the reality of that every day. After each seminar, I'd retreat to my room on campus and pass out face down on the bed all afternoon. As the week and a half went on, the deleterious effects became cumulative, and I could hardly draw myself out of bed to dress for class and strike out across the snowy campus in the frigid, late February air.

My hands were the most afflicted at this time. I stumbled to button my shirts as pain beat like a metronome through my knuckles; it radiated into my palms so that my entire hand was clenched like a throbbing claw. I slathered my hands in natural arthritis-relieving arnica cream and hoped that it would give me a few hours of relief in the classroom. I gulped coffee before class with the faith that it would provide me with just enough energy to lecture and lead discussions.

The students and Professor Newport never knew that week how much I struggled, as my pride would not allow me to mention my symptoms or my fatigue, but when I flew back to Houston at the end of the seminar, the Lyme flare-up threw me down into bed. I could not rise up against climate change.

The Summer of 2017: My Full-Time Protocol

I ramped up my protocol in 2017. To combat the aggressive, thinly coiled spirochetes, I swallowed a mountain of organic supplements and herbs throughout the day. I self-prescribed oregano oil, garlic, cat's claw, wormwood, and caprylic acid.

The anti-handyman who was my husband built a far infrared sauna in our basement that was supposed to relieve joint pain and kill spirochetes. It made me feel nauseous, which seemed to indicate it was having some effect, but I couldn't chart any improvement in my symptoms.

When I wasn't in the sauna, I was lying on an amethyst BioMat, filled with coils that convert electricity into far infrared rays. The heat is said to alleviate arthritic symptoms and fatigue. The BioMat sucked out my pain while I was lying on it, but the effects were temporary.

I also tried a Rife machine, a device created by Raymond Rife that generates radio frequencies meant to kill off bacteria, viruses, and cancer cells. Rife machines hold a certain mythological value for Lyme sufferers, since some patients vow to have been cured by them. Dr. Phillips didn't officially advocate for the use of Rife machines, but back when I first became his patient in 2014, he shared that some patients had found them helpful. He remained neutral, since, as he writes in his recent book *Chronic*, "there is no published data specifically proving efficacy for the treatment of Lyme," but he knew that I was using it.[4] In the afternoons, I fastened the Velcro electrodes of my Rife machine to the palms of my hands and the soles of my feet. I set the frequencies on the digital control box to cycle through the nine Lyme settings that my manual indicated while I lay on the BioMat.

Equally famous to Lyme patients are the Jarisch-Herxheimer reactions that Rife machines can spur on. A "herx" is the body's violent reaction to endotoxin-like waste being released as the spirochetal organisms die off in the body. Dr. Phillips had warned me years ago that I would herx on our aggressive antibiotic treatment, saying "some Herxheimer reactions make people so sick they feel like they're dying." The sudden and extreme die-off exacerbates Lyme symptoms as the body struggles to detoxify at such a rapid rate.

Attached to the Rife machine, I'd feel the pulsating current travel through my body and shiver for forty-five minutes. When I undid the electrodes and wires and went to stand up, I'd fall on the floor, dizzy. But it never eradicated my symptoms.

Then, if I could muster the energy to get there, I'd float in the salt-water pool—which we had converted from chlorine in the hope that the salt would have some therapeutic effects on me—as a reward for enduring these questionable methodologies.

In spite of all these failed attempts to get well, I believed in positive affirmations, and I repeated them every single day, no matter how dead I felt. *I will be well. I will be well.*

2

THE ALTERNATIVE WAS ASSISTED SUICIDE

In illness . . . we cease to be soldiers in the army
of the upright. We become deserters.

—Virginia Woolf, *On Being Ill*

Over the years, Lyme had sucked the marrow out of me and spat me out like an enervated double of my old self. I could no longer endure the Sisyphean battle of waking up feeling depleted, hardly able to struggle through the most basic tasks, only to have to repeat the cycle the next day. There was no high-level thinking. I couldn't play my musical instruments. I had no positive energy to share with my friends, so I stopped seeing them. I couldn't hightail it along hiking trails. I had the heart and mind of a teacher, but I had no students to teach, and what's worse, I couldn't retain an idea long enough to teach it.

In late 2016, I experienced a brief reprieve. I'd lost my grandmother and my beloved Brady, and, in the vortex of that grief, my body allowed me a mysterious burst of energy, perhaps as a consolation. I hiked my sadness off in Patagonia, fueled by the adrenaline of mourning, astonished at my body's ability. But then, only a few months later, I fell ill again. I had become accustomed to riding the unpredictable roller coaster of what Lyme doctors and fellow patients refer to as the "new normal," but this low felt the worst. Things just started falling apart in my body, more than ever before. Inexorably, gravity pulled me to the bed, and I stayed there for months.

I had constant joint pain, and my cognitive issues worsened to the extent that I couldn't read more than a short text message. I resided in a permanent stupor. Even changing a lightbulb seemed like a staggering task. Tinnitus and sinusitis were omnipresent, so even when I was resting in bed, my ears were ringing and my nasal passages were painfully blocked.

New symptoms cropped up too. I'd wake up with wet hair, a soaking nightgown, and drenched skin from mysterious night sweats. "I'm dressed in summer like I'm going skiing," D—Dmitri's nickname—complained, when he had to wear base layers and long johns to bed because I had the air conditioning set to 66 degrees. (And believe me, as an environmentalist, setting the thermostat there wasn't done lightly.)

"But I'm burning up, D," I whimpered back.

He nodded with waning pity.

My heart started having wild improv sessions in my chest, waking me up in the night with its fast beats and syncopated rhythms. The doctors had told me that tachycardia, or increased heart rate with abnormal beats, was yet another symptom of chronic Lyme disease. *Would I have a heart attack as a result of Lyme?*

For an introductory talk at a poetry reading my nonprofit was hosting at Pen and Brush in New York City, I had to write down every word I planned to say, and no one knew what it cost me to get there. My childhood friend Doug tried to be helpful afterward, saying, "We need to get you off the written page more."

"But I couldn't remember my thoughts for a minute," I said.

He nodded blankly. No one seemed to understand, even my old besties. The poet Meghan O'Rourke suffers from late-stage neurological Lyme, and her poem "How to Be" mirrors how I felt: "like a person whose language has slipped away."[1] I had no language, and I had no home in my own mind.

One day, Dmitri's collaborator on a new project knocked on the door before he arrived home, and I shuddered when I looked in the mirror on my way to the door. I greeted her in old UGG slippers, baggy plaid lavender pajama pants with a hole in the right knee, a moth-eaten turquoise cardigan, dirty hair wound up in a bun, and a pair of smudged, old glasses. It was the middle of the afternoon. I tried to imagine what she was seeing when I ushered her in. The foyer looked like hoarders had taken up residence.

"I'm mortified," I repeated when I gestured to myself, my home, my forgetfulness.

"Michelle, it's fine. This is real life. I get to see the real you," she said.

"This is not the real me, I promise you," I said, but I could see that she didn't believe me. I had to sit with her in my ill-person uniform until Dmitri arrived, stripped of my last vestige of dignity. "I can't do this anymore," I said to the mirror after she left. "I can't do this anymore," I told D out loud that night.

We had scheduled a trip to London for summer, but now I begged him to go without me. His well of energy was drying up from taking care of me, and it pained me to see that I was depleting him too. He went, and while he was dancing with our friends at an indie rock festival in Hyde Park, I was lying in bed in the middle of the day.

It was a Saturday in early July. Desperate and immobilized, I clutched my phone and launched my millionth Google search for answers. Variations of "cure+chronic+late-stage+neurological+Lyme disease" featured in my frantic searches—conducted late at night when the joint pain in my hands and feet woke me up—and I often cried at the paucity of solutions.

Research is what I had done best in my previous life, but my brain couldn't focus on words and paragraphs anymore. When I had respites from the pain, I'd log on to the Johns Hopkins online library to read medical research on Lyme disease, autoimmune disorders, heavy metal toxicity, mold toxicity, and cures. I became an expert medical researcher, but my research wasn't curing me. I had been in bed for months, since early March.

As I had all summer, I was wearing long sleeves that day to hide the reptilian patches of psoriasis on my arms and the candida rashes I had developed. Even though I was alone, I couldn't bear to see the sores. Psoriasis is an autoimmune disorder, its presence evidence of my immune system's inability to ward off invaders. As a side effect of Lyme medications, I had a raging case of candida, so I googled "candida cures."

Like following a chain of signifiers, I came to a passage on a forum called Cure Zone, which referred in a reverent way to a Dr. Filonov. Uncomfortable on my back with my head propped on pillows, I made a micro-turn to curl into my right side and wedge a pillow between my aching knees. Sighing in discomfort from the move, thirsty, but unable to make the round trip to the kitchen and back to bed, I continued to read.

Dr. Filonov purportedly cured patients through extreme fasting methods that "incinerated diseased cells in the body" and "drained the swamp of inflammation."

I read, "According to Siberian doctor Sergey Filonov, dry fasting activates each cell to become an incinerator and burn bacteria and viruses in the body; when deprived of water, inflammation is eliminated." I put the phone down on my duvet and stared at my bedroom in wonder. *Incinerate diseases.* The flood of incoming thoughts about the implications instigated another bout of tachycardia.

But this was one of the most intriguing sentences I had ever read. I was inflamed, and I was harboring much that needed to be burned in my body. I reached for my phone and tapped a flurry of searches to find this mythical-sounding Dr. Filonov, but he eluded me.

I switched my iPhone keyboard over to Russian and spelled out Филинов. Having a Russian-born husband and a lifelong interest in Russian literature and music, I could read haltingly in the Russian language.

The linguistic switch yielded access to Dr. Filonov's site, but I couldn't wield the phone any longer; my hands were throbbing from cradling it. The tinnitus rose in a strident crescendo in my ears. My eyes hurt looking at the screen and I kept blinking to focus. I wanted to learn more but I had to put the phone down and pause for a nap.

• • •

When I woke up a few hours later, I learned that the radical treatment Dr. Filonov espoused consisted of dry fasting—or refraining from eating or drinking anything, including water—for a period of time. The site said he cured diseases with extended dry fasts of nine days or more. One started incrementally with a thirty-six-hour dry fast, from, say, seven p.m. on a Saturday to seven a.m. on Monday. I was copying passages into Google Translate, since I had exceeded my capacity to interpret Russian instructions. He described an elaborate preparatory protocol that should take place over a period of months, involving progressively longer water fasts. I didn't have a month, though.

A few weeks before, I'd met my childhood friend Kate at a restaurant in Chelsea. It hurt to go—literally, it was hard to sit in a restaurant chair—but I wanted to see her. "Kate," I said, "I'm at the end of my ability to fight. I'm planning to commit assisted suicide."

She reached across the table to hold my hand for a moment. "Miche, will you please let me know when it's time, so I can have a chance to say goodbye?" she asked. Though I could hardly sit up, I held her gaze and nodded. I appreciated that she wasn't trying to talk me out of it.

Kate had watched me wane away over the last several years. We'd been friends since we were girls at Interlochen. If anyone knew that this "new normal" wasn't me, it was her. I had lost my Micheness, my identity, my way of showing up in the world, and Kate loved me enough to be able to let me go. We both knew that a part of me had already died, thanks to Lyme.

I had read the results of a study by the British think tank Demos on the link between suicide and chronic illness. Ten percent of suicides in the U.K. are attributed to an inability to tolerate chronic illness; one person with a chronic illness commits suicide a day in the United Kingdom.[2]

As I'd been investigating Dr. Filonov's site, D had been sending photos of our friends dancing at The Killers concert. The contrast between their gaiety and my moribund state deepened my sense of despair.

Although I still felt "lovable as is," my new mantra, I couldn't see through dense brain fog. It was no longer enough to have compassion for myself, to accept myself as I was. I couldn't move. I couldn't go on.

I had read every health study, every health book, every medical journal. I had experimented on my own body as if I were a laboratory animal. I had exhausted every known and unknown treatment. I had nothing left to try.

I began my first dry fast that Saturday afternoon in early July. I didn't tell anyone. With my intermittent napping, I barely noticed I hadn't had water until it was past my bedtime. By the middle of the night, I grew increasingly thirsty and weak. Dizzy and not trusting myself to walk, I crawled to the bathroom. To my surprise, I urinated multiple times, even though I hadn't taken a sip of water for hours. I was in a desert delirium by morning, but I did not yield to the thirst. *Incinerate, cells. Burn the Lyme away*, I whispered to my body. When I reached twenty-four hours, on late Sunday afternoon, I sloshed water down my face and into my mouth like a dog lapping from a bowl of water in the heat of summer. Spent.

I crawled back to bed weaker than ever, thinking, *But I am still alive. I don't want to commit suicide and leave the world enervated like this*. I was determined to contact Dr. Filonov and become his patient.

3

CONVINCING D

If only D would call him on my behalf, I thought, *he could explain my case in Russian, but he will have to be convinced.* I had two more days until D was to come home. I closed my eyes and rummaged for the origin story I would narrate for Dr. Filonov.

I never thought I would be debilitated from a serious illness, because I had always been dubbed a "health nut." I became a vegetarian when I was a teenager. I have been a lifelong evangelist for organic vegetables and fruits, to the amusement of my friends and family. I have meditated and practiced yoga since I was a teenager. I started hiking solo on the Long Trail in Vermont when I was fifteen, and I had skied and run marathons for years. I had always been a fierce proponent of self-care on psychological, spiritual, and physical levels. How could I have become someone who lived in her bed?

I had practiced nutritional experiments on myself and on my open-minded father and friends since I was a child. My father and I were always exceptionally close, but after my mother died when I was a young teenager, he allowed me to be his amateur nutritionist. When we were strictly macrobiotic, Dad protested breakfasts of seaweed mixed with steamed vegetables and brown rice, but he appreciated the newfound energy it brought us. When we were raw vegan, Dad exclaimed that he could wear his trousers from college, and he needed far less sleep. When I started a lifelong practice of green juice fasting at the age of seventeen, Dad implemented a weekly day of juice or water fasting day that he still practices. He was also my confidant when my health took an inexplicable turn years before.

I now think this was likely when I first contracted Lyme, though I had no idea at the time. It was 2005, and I was studying for my doctoral degree at Johns Hopkins. Seemingly from nowhere, I developed alarming symptoms. I needed my high-functioning brain to write my dissertation, but I stopped thinking clearly, and I needed to take naps for the first time since early childhood. I confided in my dad.

"Dad, my brain is the only thing I care about. I can't speed-read or retain details anymore. I'm rereading paragraphs, and I still can't remember them. Something is wrong. What if I get kicked out of Hopkins?" I agonized.

"We will find help for you. No, of course I'm not going to tell anyone about this. Don't worry." Dad was reassuring, but I could tell he was flummoxed, too.

In spite of these mysterious symptoms, my will was strong, my discipline was indefatigable. I rose every single day at 4:45 a.m. to write my dissertation, until I defended it successfully. Since I was able to function on such a high level, I didn't take the symptoms seriously, and the fatigue receded again.

But when I started a tenure-track position in Wisconsin, I'd collapse after each day's work. It took me far longer than usual to grade essays and prepare lectures and lesson plans. I was waking up at five in the morning and going to sleep at midnight in order to keep up with my academic workload. Nothing seemed to alleviate the fatigue, so I had to quit.

In the summer of 2012, I went to Istanbul for a comparative literature conference, where something took over my body and mind. While my colleagues were exploring Turkey on the weekends, I was sleeping in my hotel room. I developed excruciating pain in my joints that I could almost hear out loud. I learned the definition of migraine headache firsthand—a pain I'd never understood until then. I would sit down to edit a book I was writing, but to my dismay, I could not remember words or write in complete sentences.

When I returned to New York, I had to cancel most of the fall classes I was scheduled to teach at a local university. I spent weeks on the sofa, freezing. An abstract for a conference proposal was rejected, a devastating thing that hadn't happened to me for several years. My academic career was in shambles along with my self-esteem—and my body.

That had led to my diagnosis of Lyme disease and, with it, the advice that I learn to accept this "new normal." Except that it didn't feel anything like normal.

A couple of years passed, and D's inability to cope with a broken wife led us to a painful estrangement. During this period, I was home alone with my dog Brady for several months. Barely able to walk, let alone wield a leash with an active German shepherd at the other end, I had to hire a part-time nurse. Anthony ("Ann-toe-knee") made me garlic soup and fresh-squeezed grapefruit juice. He'd shuck oysters so that I would have extra B12. He fluttered around the house with gusto, tending to me and Brady. When nurse Anthony wasn't there, I had to do the unthinkable: ask for help.

Everyone mobilized. My friend Doug was coming up from New York on the weekends. He would make butternut squash soup for us.

We sat under blankets and watched old movies like *The Philadelphia Story* until the pain battered my head and eyes again. When he saw that I still couldn't walk or think, he said, "The shipment of hope just didn't come in today." My friend Pasha came from Greenwich and walked Brady when I was in a bind, even though he was allergic to dogs. Doug's mother, Carolyn, flew in from Toronto and stayed with us for a week. Susan drove down from Boston to bring me her homemade Thai soup, entertaining me with memories of our days at Dartmouth. Susan took Brady on such fulfilling walks that he slept on her bed at night. Cara came up whenever she could from Brooklyn, bringing the Iris Murdoch novels she used to talk about in grad school. I'd doze off, and Cara would start reading again when I woke up. Arthur came down from Vermont and planted garlic in my garden, doted on Brady, and played nocturnes on the piano. When Jim, an older, conservative friend drove down from Vermont, I couldn't even walk from my bed to the toilet. He would help me stand and walk from my bedroom to the bathroom, deposit me there, wait outside the door, then come back to make the return trip with me. Jim was a music critic, and I had frequently accompanied him to performances in my concert attire. This time, I meekly stayed in pajamas and surrendered all my standards, one by one, along with my New England stoicism.

In *On Being Ill*, Virginia Woolf writes that illness reduces self-consciousness, but I disagree. Other than requesting help from my closest friends, I sequestered myself. Being ill didn't reduce my mortification at living in flannel pajamas and sliding down the stairs on my bum.

I would feel better for a time, and think I could take a road trip, or work on my interminable academic manuscript, or travel. Then I'd fall even lower, without realizing that I was in a perilous pattern of building and burning reserves. These vicissitudes ruled my life until the great flare-up of 2017. The new normal was oppressive. More than that, it was unlivable. This is what I planned to tell Dr. Filonov.

When D returned home from London, I had a speech prepared. Over the past two days, I'd typed a letter to the doctor, detailing each stage of my nightmare. I feared that D would refuse to help me contact the doctor. D was the sort of person who would chase me around the house each time I vegetable juice-fasted, saying, "You will die if you don't eat something!" He had grown up in the Soviet Union standing in line for bread and milk as a child and, consequently, maintained a deep-seated fear of starvation. If D thought juice fasting was extreme, I could only imagine how opposed he'd be to a treatment that involved no food and no water for extensive periods.

"I'll do it," he said before I'd gotten very far into my speech. In spite of his jet lag, D translated the letter I had written. "Very good, but he doesn't need to have an encyclopedic knowledge of your medical history. He doesn't need to know that your mother breastfed you. We need to give him the *bottom line*." He paused and flung his hand out as if he were a conductor cuing me. "You're dying from Lyme disease." I marveled at how my reserved husband was throwing himself into this dubitable project. *He* was editing *me*, to my delight.

"I'm going to go to work early tomorrow. I'll make a cup of tea, settle in at my desk with a pad of paper, and then I'll call the doctor. It should be eleven or twelve hours ahead in Siberia." He kept repeating that he was going to make a cup of Earl Grey tea first, as if he was counting on the comforting warm beverage to give him the courage to make the call.

The next morning, I woke up to the ringing phone. "You need to go to Siberia now! Can you go this week?" he shouted. In my early morning Lyme fog, I had no idea what he was talking about. As a sick person whose permanent address had been 1 Bed Avenue, panic took hold of my shoulders and my chest. My bed was the only place in the world that brought me solace and when I left it, I felt like I was going into exile. D's words made the abstract idea of Siberia morph into an immediate reality. *I haven't cobbled the tax documents together yet. I committed to peer review that Cixous article. I promised Helen we would dog-sit her puppy, Albus*, I thought all at once.

"What? Wait. Deeee, I'm not ready. What did he say?" I said haltingly.

D summarized his conversation with the doctor. Dr. Filonov was not enthusiastic about taking a very sick American patient. He thought it was risky and warned D that it would be challenging to treat me, because of the vast quantity of pharmaceutical drugs I'd consumed over the past several years. "Her liver is very toxic," he repeated to D several times. D begged him to take me as a patient. "I told him several times, 'She is very motivated and determined to get well!'" D recounted.

"*Harasho*. Good. She needs to come for two months, as soon as possible, while it is still summer in Siberia," Dr. Filonov responded. D assured the doctor that I would make the journey right away.

I was hyperventilating from inner turbulence. Part of me was dumbfounded that D was so supportive. Another part of me was elated at the prospect of finding a cure. And still another part of me was terrified about leaving the safe haven of my bed. But, most of all, what I felt was skittish with hope.

4

PREPARING TO STARVE AND CONVINCING THE SKEPTICS

Those who walk on well-trodden paths always throw stones at those who are showing a new road.

—Voltaire, *The Philosophical Dictionary*

It was an arduous path to prepare for the trip. My passport was on the verge of expiring, so I got a new one. Then, with the new passport in hand, I discovered that applying for a long-term Russian visa is a byzantine process with hurdles that would deter the most determined world travelers from crossing the Russian border. All these bureaucratic procedures took time.

The preparatory protocol exhausted me even further. After D's conversation with the doctor, he used the dictionary to translate the Russian words he didn't know into English. Dr. Filonov wanted me to take one teaspoon of aluminum-free baking soda in a cup of hot water every morning for two weeks, and I was to take two tablets of "coal" on an empty stomach twice a day.

"Coal, D? That can't be right. Could it possibly be activated charcoal?" Since the Russian word implied absorbing toxins, we opted for the charcoal.

Abstemiousness followed. I gazed wistfully at my French press each morning, but I stopped drinking coffee. Coffee is an elixir that brings morning hope to the chronically ill, each sip like a jumper cable revving me into a state of wakefulness. Without it, I was tense by the end of the day from trying to keep myself glued together, but I ceased having my evening glass of red wine. I didn't veer from the ascetic path.

I relinquished my status as head doctor and turned myself over to Dr. Filonov. I stopped taking all allopathic drugs including antibiotics and the Ambien I had taken for Lyme insomnia. I maintained a plant-based organic diet consisting of homemade vegetable broth, green vegetables, and whole grains such as millet and buckwheat porridge. I juiced vegetables and added a few pumpkin and hemp seeds to my salads. I cared for the ailing vehicle of my body—as I had always done through diet—yet this strict regime brought me no relief from my Lyme symptoms. When I consulted with a naturopath in New York City, Dr. Anthony Salzarulo, he counseled me against dry fasting, but he said he remained open-minded.

I threw out all my makeup, and I stopped getting manicures and pedicures because of the formaldehyde used in nail polish and nail polish remover. I stopped wearing deodorant with aluminum—a heavy metal—so I was getting a bit stinky. Over those remaining weeks of summer, D watched me with curiosity, appreciating my disciplined approach. He couldn't resist making jokes, though, even when they were about things he didn't really understand, like what a hippie was: "You have always eaten hippie food, and worn hippie Birkenstocks, but now you smell like a hippie too."

If being an anti-chemical hippie meant that I took Rachel Carson's predictions in *Silent Spring* seriously, then I was one. The increased use of pesticides, coupled with warmer temperatures, created perfect conditions for the disease that had invaded my body. Pesticide use has led to an alarming decline of pollinators like bees. This has coincided with the significant rise of arthropods like ticks, which spread the most prevalent vector-borne disease: Lyme. Did I agree with Carson that the 600 million pounds of pesticides the U.S. government was producing back in 1960 would have dire consequences on animals and humans? Yes, I would wear my hippie label proudly in the name of healing.

When I called Dad to explain that I was going to Siberia to spend two months with Dr. Filonov, he boomed out in his authoritative lawyer's voice, "I assume Dmitri asked the primary question, 'How many people have died while undergoing your treatment?'"

"He did not ask him that, Dad," I responded. "Dr. Filonov is a respected doctor. He has not been carried off to the gulag for killing patients."

"I want Dmitri to ask him how many patients have died."

I didn't reply.

"If you insist on going, I want you to send messages to us daily."

Meanwhile, my stepmother, Janet, was keen about the Siberian venture. "Michael, she has nothing to lose. I say, go for it," I heard her say as I argued with my father on speakerphone.

"Dad, please have faith in Dr. Filonov. I'm putting my life into his hands," I pleaded.

He had always supported me in my endeavors; he was a professional dad. "I will support you," he said. The resonance of his voice carried over the phone.

After two short preparatory water fasts, I embarked on a three-day dry fast, while D was away on business. What fueled me when food and water didn't was what I had read on Dr. Filonov's site: "Dry fasting has colossal power to heal the body, and to enhance one's natural system of immunity."

The process that dry fasting ignites in the body is called autophagy. And although my father fretted, I had no fear of it. The science made sense to me—and I discuss this aspect further in Part III. My body *felt* as if it were full of debris from the inflammation, which I couldn't get out. I didn't know at the time that I was missing key detox enzymes in my genetic profile, that I didn't methylate like others did. All that knowledge would come much later. Right now, I only had the intuition, that autophagy—or self-eating—was going to cure me. I had been focused on what to put in my body, not what I could take out. I didn't know that the taking out could be healing.

The first two days of dry fasting were no worse than the daily discomfort I knew so well. I alternated between lying in the hammock, staring out at the pond, or curling up in bed. Whole weeks and months had been lost to me, so two days felt insignificant. But by the afternoon of the third day, the dryness of my tongue irritated me. I rinsed my mouth with water and spit it out, careful not to swallow a drop. Later, I'd learn why this was forbidden: it's much harder to dry fast if one comes in contact with water because it makes the mouth even dryer. When I examined myself in the mirror on the afternoon of the third day, I thought that I looked deranged. My skin had a grayish pallor, and my eyes were drooping, lifeless.

Counting down the final hours was like living life in a slow-motion movie about torture. It was more about discomfort than true pain. On the third day, about seventy-one hours into this experiment, I carefully set out a cup of hot water, a glass of cold water, and even a glass of freshly squeezed organic pink grapefruit juice. I wasn't sure which one I was supposed to have, so I planned to try all three. I had enough discipline to take a shower and don a bathrobe before I sat down to my water at the dining room table.

Tears streamed down my face in relief as the first sip of hot water seeped into my dry mouth. There was nothing to swallow, for it had all been absorbed by my eager tongue and gums, so I greedily took another, and another, until I felt satiated.

The grapefruit juice, by contrast, made me nauseous. I would learn later that citrus is forbidden during the first few days. There was no room for error in Dr. Filonov's precise exit instructions, which I hadn't yet been given.

I thought that drinking the water would put an end to my arid misery, but after imbibing liquids to rehydrate over the next few days, I was afflicted with waves of nausea, fatigue, and headaches. The lymph nodes on the roof of my mouth swelled up the way they had when I first felt acutely ill from Lyme. For over a week, I rested in bed, feeling even more obliterated than usual. I sent messages to Dr. Filonov on WhatsApp through Google Translate.

"Normal." Dr. Filonov's laconic, terse messages in Russian were challenging to interpret. He seemed to be telling me that there was no elegant way to clear the body of detritus after years of illness; I extrapolated that the hot water was carrying cellular debris out of my body at a rapid clip.

I marveled that I had access to Dr. Filonov at all, that he didn't charge me for these messages, for these mini-consultations. *How is it possible that he counsels me for free in the twenty-first century after I have spent thousands of dollars on out-of-pocket Lyme treatments?* Dmitri's mother had sent a small wire transfer from her Russian account to Dr. Filonov's, and we would be bringing the remainder of the payment in cash. Fifty dollars a day was a pittance in comparison with the cost of alternative treatments we had already covered outside of health insurance's range. This tiny figure would become increasingly astonishing to me.

• • •

I had put all my remaining hope in Dr. Filonov, so I was not dissuaded by the recovery from the fast, and neither was Dmitri. Others in my inner circle were not convinced.

I remember a couple of weeks before when I casually mentioned to my friend Helen that I was going to Siberia for this dry-fasting treatment. Like me, Helen had a Ph.D., along with a scientific mind.

"Michelle, this is *ridiculous*." She drew out the word "ridiculous." "The human body cannot *survive* for more than three days without water. Your organs will shut down. You could have *permanent damage*."

I must have rolled my eyes or averted them, because she protested.

"The human body is comprised of at least 60 percent water. Every cell needs water to function properly. I do *not* support you," she said.

Helen sent me a link to an article that I had already read, written by a man with spurious credentials, who had been sued multiple times as director of a water-fasting treatment center abroad. He argued that dry fasting was dangerous and would lead to death if attempted.

When my father referenced the same article that Helen had read, I denounced it. "Dad, Dr. Filonov has been conducting medical fasts for over thirty years. He has written books on the subject, and patients flock to him in Siberia. This is not a New Age treatment, as Helen calls it. We must trust him." When one is chronically fatigued and ill, it is excruciating to construct an argument, but I took another stab at it. "Monumental thinkers dating back to Plato and the ancient Egyptians all espoused fasting. The greatest physician of all time,

Hippocrates, wrote that our food should be our medicine but that to eat when we are sick is to feed our illness. Plutarch said that fasting was the greatest remedy and that we should fast for a day instead of relying on medicine. Even Plato said that he fasted for greater physical and mental efficiency."

"I don't doubt that these ancients fasted, but how do we know they *dry* fasted?" he countered.

We continued these conversations in person when D and I took a final trip to see Dad and Janet before we left for Siberia. We drove to Vermont with Helen's gigantic Komondor puppy, Albus, in tow with the hope that he would provide levity and distraction for the visit.

There was something very odd about our last weekend in Vermont, but it was impossible to speak about it. When we turned into the driveway, we saw they had been watching for us from the window. Janet rushed out. Her soft red hair was neatly arranged around her face. She was wearing a linen striped shirt with white jeans and her favorite Birkenstocks.

"You have arrived, D and TOC! Our favorite people. Oh, my word, and who do we have here? Well, why don't you just look at this fine fellow?" She greeted us with hugs and pats. I was TOC; she had given me the nickname when I explained to Dad one night in a Lyme stupor that I was the only child.

"Albus, come here. Come see me!" Albus leaned against the electric wheelchair where Dad could easily pet him. "Albus," Dad said affectionately, "we'll make sure you have a very good time in Vermont." Man and dog made a gargantuan, white-haired, handsome couple, since Albus was a 150-pound Komondor puppy and Dad was a six-foot-five gentleman when measured from crown to toe.

Dad patted my head, not strong enough to move his arms, which had been afflicted with a mixture of post-polio syndrome and neuropathy. Along with his sharp mind, Dad had the blood pressure of an athlete, though. "Oh, my beautiful Michelley, am I ever so happy to see you," he said, shining his blue eyes at me.

I crashed on the sofa under a forget-me-not-blue blanket that one of Dad's caregivers knitted for him. I always made a beeline from the car to the sofa during the Lyme years. Everyone crowded around me, as if they were afraid there would never be another chance to converse. Janet made my favorite soup that we called my "sick soup," with simple vegetables and water. Dad stationed himself by my side.

Dmitri scoured the farmer's market and cooked all their favorite foods with exaggerated gusto, generated perhaps by a nervousness he didn't know how to articulate. He explained to Dad and Janet over and over that he would fly with me all the way to Siberia, drive me to the clinic, make sure I was settled, and then continue on to Singapore on business. This seemed to reassure them.

The palms of my afflicted hands and the soles of my feet throbbed so loudly I could barely focus on the conversation, but I refused to mention it that weekend; we had discussed my pain ad nauseam. Virginia Woolf writes that "we must invent language to describe pain," and I agree with her about describing one's pain, but I also agree with the philosopher Ludwig Wittgenstein, who insists that we cannot know another's pain.[1] D had heard my linguistic inventions surrounding pain for years, but my descriptions never endowed him with the empathetic ability to fully understand it. My family could only acknowledge my pain, which they had done to the point of exhaustion.

She didn't voice it then, but inwardly, Janet was concerned about a dreadful winter coming on early in Siberia, and she even entertained thoughts of the political tensions between our countries causing trouble for me. Dad was blunt about his serious reservations.

"I recall the IRA hunger strikes of years ago, where each guy on strike succumbed after about twenty-five days without food, but with water. This adventure you're going on in Siberia without food or water is giving rise to substantial concerns about your participation." He paused before continuing. "You still have not given me an answer to the question as to how many patients have died while undergoing this, er, treatment." At the word "treatment," he seemed to choke.

I looked over at Dad with newfound sympathy, realizing that from his perspective, I—the only child—was going to a place that he associated with hardship, to undergo a treatment that seemed dangerous. "I love you, Daddy," I whispered. It was a term I hadn't brought out in years, and he nodded back at me with an expression in his bright blue eyes that I understood: pain mixed with love. I had their tenuous blessing.

5

BOUND FOR THE LAND OF GULAGS AND PERMAFROST

Siberia has traditionally been associated with cold, darkness, prisons, and wild nature. . . . A stereotypical picture prevails: a vast land where distance separates people and where isolation has affected people's mental state, a wild country with impenetrable forests and blizzardy tundra inhabited in most part by wolf packs, a destination for deportations.

—**Aivar Jürgenson,** "The Formation of Siberian Identity and One of Its Political Manifestations"

It was mid-August when, paperwork finally in place, Dmitri and I were able to fly to Siberia. We had a late evening flight, and by early evening I could hardly get out of bed to go to the taxi. Curled in my yoga pants like a fiddlehead fern, I had clenched my eyes closed. I folded my hands into my chest, as pain hammered into my knees, feet, back, and hands like a persistent drill. D turned on the bedroom light—it seemed to blare—and came and stood over me. "Are you sure you can make this trip? I'm not sure we can handle this. What do you think?" He spoke in an anxious tone that sounded like shouting, but my volume button had been broken for a long time—all sounds were freakishly amplified in my Lyme-ridden brain.

"The taxi is downstairs, and we need to make a decision," he said. He sounded tense, scared, and I could tell he was considering whether we should call off Project Siberia.

I knew I had to rally, or else I would never rise up again. I did not want to commit assisted suicide.

"Just carry me to the car," I pleaded, eyes still closed. He put one more pair of warm socks in the suitcase, muttering, "Her feet will get cold in Siberia." D zipped the case up. The crisp zipping sound seemed dramatic and final to me. I had surrendered the final packing to the most disorganized person I knew. I realized I was going far, far away, and I wasn't even sure what was in my suitcase. This was really happening. We were going to Siberia.

Once we had gotten my body out of the taxi and through security at John F. Kennedy airport, it was nearly midnight. Mustering all my strength to remain upright in the unforgiving metal chair as we waited to board, I longed for the safety of my bed. "Mmmmmmm," I whimpered and then realized the sounds were audible.

I stared at my boarding pass. This tangible piece of paper with my name on it and the city of our final destination on the Siberian-Mongolian border rendered my immediate future very real. My nervous laughter must have been infectious, because D quipped, "Where are you going on vacation? 'Oh, I'm going to Siberia. To starve. As one does.'" In my sleepiness and bodily discomfort, I let out another staccato stream of giggles. It was as if I had opened a valve on a metaphorical pressure cooker that released the apprehension from my chest.

. . .

When I woke up on the plane, it was morning, and D was still sleeping, slack-jawed, so I reached for my journal to record my thoughts:

> My mother died when she was forty-two. I am forty-two. I have long feared dying at this symbolic age. I do not want to die. I want to live the full life that I have imagined for myself. I just woke up on an Aeroflot plane destined for Moscow. I slept wonderfully, after a week of fitful tossing as I wondered, "Am I deranged for going to Siberia for two months?" I feel full of toxic sludge. Siberia, here I come. I am ready to slough off the sludge and be fully alive.

When we reached the departure gate in Moscow—after a lengthy wait in the terminal—D wanted to capture an image of me, so I held up my boarding pass in front of the sign that read "Barnaul" and gave a closed-mouth smile. When he showed it to me, I looked at my yoga pants, white fleece jacket, periwinkle scarf, and unkempt blond hair. *Bedraggled. No, that's me, lovable as is*, I reminded myself.

I tried to sleep on the five-hour flight, but I kept wondering what otherness lay before me. The mere word "Siberia" struck terror in much of the world. When I said "Siberia," I thought: "gulag," "work-camp," "Stalin," "suffering," "cold," and "barrenness." The antithesis of cozy, none of these associations matched with dear old bed. *1 Bed Avenue is so far away, and I might never see it again*, I thought plaintively.

Once we reached Barnaul at dawn the following day, D retrieved my hard-plastic purple suitcase at baggage claim. I shuffled out behind him into the cool, sunlit parking lot. D handed a wad of rubles to a man standing next to a dirty sports utility vehicle. D had found him online the week before and arranged for a car rental, for there was nothing remotely resembling a car rental agency at the airport. I was impressed by his foresight. D settled me into the front passenger seat, and I just about collapsed into it. *I am headed for Dr. Filonov. I am on my way to healing*, I thought. *Just hold on a little longer.*

...

Barnaul looked charming as we headed out of town for the mountains. There was a typical domed cathedral on a grassy hillside as we turned onto the interstate. Everything struck me as hilarious at this point, and I let out another trickle of giggles when I tried sounding out the words, "I am in Siberia."

For hours, D navigated the wild Siberian roads that would lead us to Dr. Filonov's clinic in the Altai mountains. The interstate was in surprisingly fine condition, but he was not prepared for the perilous Siberian driving style. Drivers passed one another at breakneck speeds, shifting back into their own lanes just meters away from careening into our car.

D looked nearly as pale as I did by the time we stopped for lunch at a primitive café in a small town off the interstate. Plainly dressed *babushkas*, or Russian grandmothers, were serving coleslaw, borscht, and a Russian dumpling called *pelmeni*. I couldn't sit up in the café for more than a few bites of coleslaw before I had to stumble back to the car.

We continued to drive. The mountains grew taller, and there was a wide, turquoise river gushing along the interstate, glistening in the Siberian summer sun. We stopped for a moment to take a respite by its formidable banks and hug one another, knowing that we'd soon be saying farewell.

As we neared the village of Ust-Sema, which we had plugged into Google Maps, it was nearly impossible to find the doctor's center. I had thought that we'd be able to stop and ask, "Where is Dr. Filonov's clinic?" I thought everyone would know where it was and that they'd be proud of their famous doctor. D started stopping and asking people selling homemade honey on the side of the road where we could find Dr. Filonov, but no one had heard of him.

D then called the doctor's daughter, Anastasia, over WhatsApp. She told us to take a right turn at the village market, go over a bridge, and proceed left down a dirt road for several kilometers, and then we'd find it.

Notoriously hopeless with directions, D found the pine-lined dirt road that brought us to a closed iron gate in a field. It seemed that we were at a dead end. D turned off the car and stared at the gate. Exasperation was rolling off him.

"I cannot believe we've traveled all the way to the heart of Siberia, and we don't have a physical address for the doctor," D said. "What are we doing?"

I ventured out of the car and stepped around the gate. As I shuffled up the path, I could see outlines of rustic wooden *dachas*, or cabins, in the distance across the field. A German shepherd puppy, its glossy coat the color of cinnamon and pepper, came running toward me.

I knew we were in the right place. In my delirium, I decided that the puppy was a definitive sign. I thought of my dog Brady, whom I still missed.

As if in a modern version of *Doctor Zhivago*, a lady in jeans and a sweatshirt with a swinging chestnut ponytail ran toward us, calling, "Nora! Nora!" I almost expected Maurice Jarre's song "Lara's Theme" to start playing in the Siberian field. She called out a greeting in Russian, "*Privyet!*" But the puppy was suspicious of me and kept barking. The lady hugged me and started speaking in Russian with a smile, "Michelle, Michelle, *ya* Valentina Filonova! Я ждала тебя." This was the doctor's wife, Valentina Filonova, and she'd been waiting for me to arrive. I was so dazed that this all made sense to me.

With the puppy, Nora, running around me and Valentina still hugging me and speaking Russian to me in a rapid sing-song tone, I gesticulated to D.

Valentina opened the big gate. He drove down the path through the field to the *dachas* that stood against a background of mountains and woods. In the distance, I heard a vivacious river. *Was it the same glacial river we had passed on the interstate?* We were in the thick of the mountains with no modern infrastructure on site. If it weren't for Valentina's jeans and sweatshirt, I would have thought we had stepped into another century altogether.

6

MEETING DR. FILONOV

We needed to wash our hands after the journey. Valentina directed us to the porch of the *bania*, where there was an orange plastic bucket hanging upside down with a spigot coming out of the bottom. It was the only faucet on site. A worn remnant of soap sat on the deck railing. We scrubbed our hands there, humbled.

Valentina showed us to a charming *dacha* that had pretty wood carvings on the overhang above the doorway. It looked like a life-sized gingerbread house. Inside, several rough-hewn twin beds were set up around a primitive wood stove. I was the only patient there; the center was between programs, and the next group of patients wouldn't be arriving until the following week. I chose a twin daybed near a window that was by the only dresser. Just behind it was a somewhat private corner where I could store my suitcase.

Valentina told us that the generator provided electricity from seven to ten p.m. every night, so I should charge my electronics accordingly.

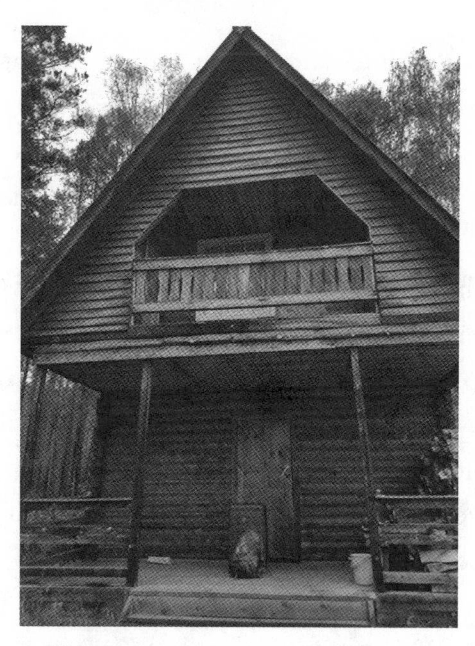

My gingerbread-house *dacha* in Siberia

D had packed external battery packs and multi-pronged chargers, having been forewarned. As she left us, giving us each a kiss on the cheek, Valentina informed D that it was an off week for staff as well, but that the doctor would be there for dinner the following evening, which also happened to be his birthday. Disappointment flooded my heart when I realized that I wouldn't be meeting Dr. Filonov right away, but it was fleeting since I was delirious with fatigue.

D spread out my massive yellow down Marmot mountaineering sleeping bag on top of the bed. Among my mountaineering sleeping bags, we had packed the heaviest one, with a lower range of minus 50 degrees Fahrenheit. Longstanding stereotypes of Siberian winters informed our decision.

Fighting jet lag, we stumbled back to the *bania*, the wooden sauna cabin where one bathes, to wash off the residue of our long journey. A roaring fireplace heated a large vat of piping hot water. D showed me how to use the basins and buckets and we each sat in the heated wooden sauna and dumped water over ourselves. When we returned to the cabin, D fell asleep as soon as he closed his eyes. I was still disoriented by the thought that he'd be leaving me the next day and couldn't sleep.

Valentina had asked D to drive her to the city of Gorno Altaisk the next morning so that she could run errands at the vegetable markets and pick up a patient from the regional airport. Tears sprung to my eyes when D told me this. "But doesn't she know that I won't see you for two months?"

He responded, simply, "This is RGO style. I can't do anything about it. I'm sorry."

RGO was one of D's famous sarcastic nicknames. Literally, it stood for Russian Gas Oil, but, in his vernacular, it was a condescending term that had many meanings. In this instance, RGO hearkened back to times of the collective in the Soviet Union, when everyone had to help out and do their part to survive. An "RGO," or Soviet, wouldn't prioritize my emotional needs—like the desire to spend every last minute with my husband before I had to begin the process of starving by myself in Siberia—over a more practical need.

Now I watched him sleep. This man cared for me enough to escort me to the end of the earth after bearing the weight of my illness for years. *Because he doesn't want to see you die from Lyme disease.* He was so tired he'd fallen asleep in his clothes and so was still dressed in jeans and a T-shirt that read, "NE 3, ATL 28 3rd 2:12."

Reading those abbreviations, which would be cryptic in Siberia, I silently repeated our mantra of 2017: *Never give up. Never, ever give up.* D had worn that T-shirt on this trip to encourage me. The winter before, we'd attended the Super Bowl just a couple of miles away from our house in Houston. At the end of the third quarter, Atlanta

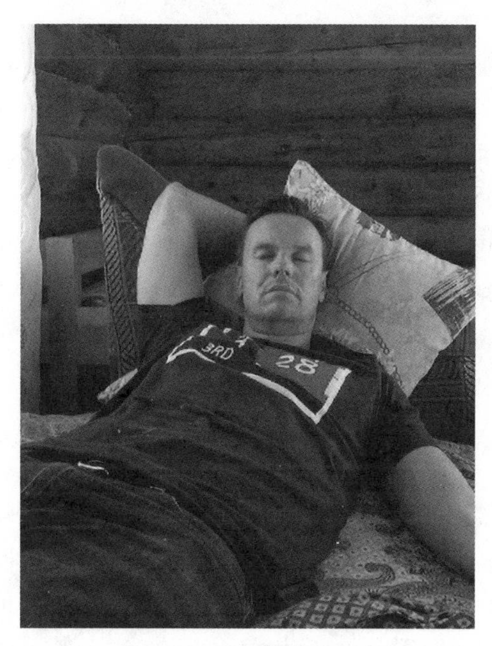

D, sleeping in his 3–28 shirt

was walloping the New England Patriots by twenty-five points for a downright humiliating score of 28–3. We held hands and when I doubted, D squeezed my hand and told me to keep steadfast faith that the Patriots would win the game. In what became the largest comeback in Super Bowl history, in the first Super Bowl overtime, the Patriots surged back—with unwavering discipline and their characteristic determination—to win the Super Bowl 34–28. Confetti fell on our heads. Fireworks illuminated the stadium. The message of D's T-shirt was this: if the Patriots could rally after such a deficit, I could rally from Lyme disease.

I had swiped my iPhone into airplane mode when we took off from New York. Not only had I read alarming articles about Russian hackers stealing personal data, but my carrier, AT&T, charged astronomical international rates. D had given me a spare Samsung phone connected to his T-Mobile account that had modest international data rates.

A feeble signal permitted me to send WhatsApp messages, but I wouldn't be able to load anything from the internet or get enough of a signal to call out most of the time. Before we'd left, D had set up a family chat called Siberia! Sweet Siberia! and I used it now to send a picture of him sleeping. Janet responded so swiftly that I realized she and my dad must have been staring at the phone, waiting for messages. "Someone is having a well-deserved rest. We love the photos. Let the work begin! Hard for us to believe you have arrived in this faraway land."

. . .

When I woke up, D had already gone on his errands. Rolling out of my cocoon, I investigated the contents of my suitcase to see what D had packed for me. This turned out to be various shirts and a sweater, but only two pairs of yoga pants and one pair of hiking pants. I had some yoga shorts, too, but I wondered how long the Siberian climate would permit me to wear them. I donned a black pair of yoga pants, a long-sleeved white T-shirt, and my purple down vest, eager to look around the clinic grounds.

The gentle Siberian sun bade me good morning. There was no humidity, a welcome discovery as humidity made my joints swell up grotesquely. There were a few more *dachas* spaced apart in the emerald grass, and a grassy path led to the central area. Pine-covered mountains rose ahead of me, and the taiga lay behind me. My body yearned to return to the sleeping bag; it resisted being upright and felt heavy. But I walked to the kitchen hut nonetheless. I passed the medical *dacha* on the left and crossed the dirt driveway to the spot where a long outdoor picnic table was covered in a roughhewn roof with open sides. *This must be where the patients eat their meals when they break their fasts*, I thought. Just to the left of the picnic table, there was a fire pit with worn wooden benches arranged in a square around it.

Embers were smoldering there. I looked up to see a valley in the distance with yet more mountains behind it, creating a panorama. Beyond the fire pit, there were wooden steps leading down to a covered landing that overlooked a small dam. A brook trickled down from the mountains and passed through the dam, just loudly enough for me to hear on the landing. I couldn't see where it went.

"доброе утро, мишель!"

I looked up and saw the cook, Lena, standing in the doorway of the kitchen hut waving at me. We had briefly met her yesterday, as she was the only staff member on site. Her cherub cheeks spread in a smile, and her wavy blond hair fell to her chin. "Good morning," I called back to her in Russian, and she gesticulated with an eating pantomime, beckoning me to come inside the wooden kitchen hut with the domed roof. It looked like the stuff fairytales were made of.

Although the morning air was warm, it was cold inside the hut. It had a cracked cement floor, and there was a bench along a wall with a small table in front of it. Straight to the back, there were two stoves that must have been connected to propane tanks. On the right, there were shelves to store food and dishes. I was impressed that it was so cool in summer, like a root cellar.

Lena put a bowl of hot buckwheat kasha on the table. She gestured for me to sit and eat my *завтрак*, or breakfast. She stirred aromatic grasses in a yellow teapot and poured a cup for me. I understood she was saying that it was Siberian herbal tea. I thought I had better eat and drink whatever they gave me while I could. Lena and I quickly reached the limit of our linguistic capacities to converse, so I focused on therapeutic chewing.

In Dr. Filonov's book on dry fasting, which I had read over the past weeks with the help of Google Translate, he urges patients to chew each bite thirty times to ensure proper digestion. This was another of his protocol guidelines that I had followed fastidiously. While I ate, I peered around, taking in the crates of cabbages, carrots, potatoes, and onions. When D returned with Valentina, there would be crates of broccoli, dill, and lettuce rounding out the mix of vegetables. Glass spice jars lined the top shelf, along with pots of the famous Siberian honey we had seen being sold alongside the roads.

I saw the Russian translation of my latest letter to Dr. Filonov sitting on the shelf. I had given it to Valentina the night before, in hopes that she would present it to Dr. Filonov before I met him. I became acutely aware of the emotional pathos that had gone into that letter, and I blushed as I chewed the earthy Russian porridge.

A large figure appeared in the doorway. "Good morning, Michelle! I am Vitali, the doctor visiting from Italy. I am apprenticing with Dr. Filonov." He stepped into the hut. With raven-black hair, shining black eyes, and glowing skin, Vitali looked like he had been doing his share of fasting as a critical part of his apprenticeship.

"I have been very excited for you come. We have been wait for your arrival. Worry about visa," Vitali said, reaching for my letter on the shelf. "I am from the former Soviet republic of Moldova, and although I have lived in Italy for a long time, Russian is my native language." As Vitali read my letter, I squirmed a bit. It hadn't occurred to me that anyone but the doctor would read it.

We discovered that French was the language we had most in common.

It still wasn't perfect, but we somehow cobbled a coherent conversation together. Not being much of a grains person, I had had enough of the porridge, and Vitali said, "Leave it! We walk to the river now."

"I'm not up for a robust walk, Vitali."

"We will walk slowly!"

I followed him behind my *dacha* and into the woods on an inconspicuous path.

The pine trees stretched into the sky. Moss and ferns lined the narrow footpath, and I could hear the river roaring behind us. I was enchanted by all of this. "Vitali, it is one of the most beautiful forests I have ever seen. I am going to be so happy here. The light is tremendous. I can feel the healing energy here!" I beamed at him.

Vitali smiled and asked if I was sure I didn't want to rent a house in the neighboring village. "I apologize for how rundown the clinic is."

"I'm very proud to be a patient of Dr. Filonov. The natural beauty makes up for the humble buildings," I assured him.

I had to sit down in the moss to rest. Vitali truly hadn't understood how weak I was. He guided me through the woods and down the embankment to the beautiful turquoise river D and I had seen the day before. He showed me a spring trickling out of the mountainside into the river, and I realized that it was the same water as that which came from the stream by the center.

"You will be filling your water bottle with the healing water here when you break the dry fasts," he said.

It was just like Patagonia, where I could drink water straight out of the mountain in the Andes with no filtration. I was in awe of it all. "I'm so grateful to be here, Vitali," I repeated.

I could barely walk another step up the path to the clinic. Another ache spot at that time was in the soles of my feet, and I could feel them crunching and throbbing in spite of my cushioned Asics running shoes. The heaviness came over me again, making me feel like I was full of mercury. I was going into full-on still-life mode. My face fell, and I couldn't return Vitali's smile this time.

"Please to keep going, Michelle," Vitali urged me.

When we reached the grass clearing again, I went straight to the *dacha* to lie down. There, I wrote some pretty pessimistic words in my journal: "I am in Siberia. My body is failing. It's just going to seed. I feel like I am full of toxic sludge and can't move. Congested. Aching. Weary." Sleep came to the rescue.

When I woke up, D was sitting on the edge of my bed. "Good afternoon," he said.

"That means it's almost time for you to go," I cried, reaching out so I could place my head in his lap.

"No, no, I don't have to leave until like ten p.m. We have plenty of time." D patted my head. "Valentina is full of energy," he said. "She dragged me to every vegetable market in Gorno Altaisk, and I told her how much you love broccoli."

I laughed.

"We picked up another patient. Natalia Chernetsova. She is very nice. Please try to make friends with her." I could hear in his voice that he was feeling more comfortable about leaving me here.

"Natasha," I said.

"That's right," D nodded. "That's the Russian short name for Natalia. Vitali wants to show us some botanical garden."

"Have you met Dr. Filonov yet?" I asked.

"No, he is supposed to come back this afternoon. We shopped for his birthday dinner, and I even got some fancy RGO wine from the Crimea." D rolled his eyes and made air quotations marks when he spoke the word "fancy." He was always full of sarcasm for his native country, although I could tell from his demeanor that he had enjoyed his excursion with Valentina.

We found Vitali sitting and reading by D's rental car. "Michelle!" He bounded up from his book when he saw me. "You did not overdo it? You are okay? I forgot how ill you are!"

I nodded, even though the heaviness was still with me. D helped me settle into the front seat, and we set off for the botanical gardens.

These lay only a short drive away, and as I wandered through them, I felt the lifelong imprinted images of Siberia break apart in my mind and float away. There were variegated flowers and trees from many parts of the world in this hidden sanctuary. I fell on them with delight, exclaiming, "Echinacea!" "Blue spruce!" "Lavender!" "Dahlias!" Green hills encircled us, populated with coniferous trees. This land was far from barren. Vitali helped us pick some healing Siberian herbal teas that were dried on site from the famous medicinal herbs that grew in the Altai mountains.

When we returned to the center, I saw a tall figure with a distinguished posture standing by the fire pit. His cropped hair was sandy blond, and he had a straight nose that almost looked Native American. I knew at once that it was Dr. Filonov. As we parked, he turned and gazed into my eyes. I stared back, struck even from afar by his calm wisdom.

Getting out of the car, I noticed his athletic figure, which looked like it had withstood much dry fasting. There was a stoicism about him that reminded me of my maternal grandfather. He started walking to the car, accompanied by Nora, who barked at me as she protected what was obviously her main human. "Мишель! Мы ждали вас! Добро пожаловать!" Dr. Filonov stepped right up to me and hugged me. His eyes were the same shade of Slavic greyish blue that Dmitri's were. I felt at home looking into them and could feel tears springing into my own. I could hear Dmitri quietly translating: "Michelle, we have been waiting for you! Welcome to Siberia!"

I beamed a very genuine smile at Dr. Filonov and said, "*Spasibo! Ochen' Priyatna, poznakomitsya!*" (Thank you! It's such an honor to meet you.) I whispered to D, "Is it *dame raz . . . dinie*?"

"No, it's *S Dnem Rozhdeniya*," D whispered back, twice so I would get it. I repeated this greeting of "happy birthday" to my doctor.

"Thank you!" he answered me in English.

Ever the efficient American, I launched right into asking him if he had read my letter and when we would get started on the treatments. I expressed all this in my broken Runglish. Dr. Filonov waved his hand away. "Tonight, we will be celebrating your arrival and my birthday," he said. I bowed my head while giving a sheepish half-smile that was intended to say, *I know—I am always getting ahead of us.*

We all gathered around Dr. Filonov at the outdoor picnic table for a simple Siberian birthday meal. Valentina had made D's favorite wild mushrooms sautéed with fresh herbs they must have chosen at the markets. Lena set out a typical Russian salad of dill, golden tomato, and cucumber, and there was a bowl of miniature wild strawberries and wild raspberries for dessert. I was surprised to see dark chunks of Russian bread on the table, along with a charcuterie plate of cheeses and salami.

I would have thought that Dr. Filonov and his staff would have been eating the same sort of "hippie" food—as D called it—that I had been eating most of my life. But this was a birthday meal, one not meant for patients. Once patients started arriving, the staff ate inside the kitchen hut, so as not to tempt them while they dry fasted. That was the last time I ever saw Dr. Filonov eat in front of a patient.

Valentina, Lena, and Dr. Filonov sipped D's Crimean wine and toasted Dr. Filonov's birthday. They had many questions for Dmitri, and there was much dialogue that I didn't understand, although Vitali translated a bit of it. I was drained of my forces, and I was content to be quiet and enjoy this earthy birthday repast.

My fellow patient, Natasha, was already dry fasting, so she stayed back in her *dacha* during the meal, but, when we moved to the fire pit, I saw a thin blond figure walking toward us. Clad in black leggings, a pink T-shirt, and glasses with a messy bun on top of her head, she looked like someone I'd be able to relax around. From her maternal smile, I could see why D had encouraged me to be friends with her. "I can already tell we're going to be friends," she said to me through him, and that sounded just fine with me because she exuded gentleness.

When it came time for Dmitri and me to say goodbye, everyone stayed and watched.

Perhaps things had really not changed much from the Soviet Union, where privacy was priced at an elusive premium. I cried into his chest, clinging to his 3–28 T-shirt, and hid my face in his embrace, as if we were alone.

"Don't be sad. They will take good care of you. I promise you. I'm proud of you for being so strong. I'm rooting for you," he said in a soft tone I was unaccustomed to, and then he released me. I wrapped my arms around myself in consolation and watched as his car disappeared down the dirt road.

PART II

STARVING TO HEAL

7

PREPARING TO FAST

A little starvation can really do more for the average sick man than can the best medicine and the best doctors.

—**Mark Twain,** "At the Appetite Cure"

I needed a task to keep my mind off D's departure. I had read in Dr. Filonov's book that it was important to sleep outside while dry fasting. Since the body isn't being nourished by an external power supply of food or water, it capitalizes on moisture in the air. Ideally, the patient should fast in a pure mountainous area rife with rivers. Mountains? Check. Rivers? Check. Check. I was determined to go all-in. Sleeping outside? Done.

It was time to recreate 1 Bed Avenue in Siberia. I gathered my orange rolled-up mountaineering mattress, my sleeping bag, and a tote bag holding my journal and random gear. I moved from the cabin to the covered wooden platform by the dam. The sun had set, and the sky had deepened to an inky blue. My mountaineering headlamp made the leaves on the trees that grew along the river look gilded. I huffed and puffed to inflate my Therm-a-Rest mattress, and I spread out my sleeping bag on top of it. I kicked off my Birks and nestled into the mummy bag that I zipped up around me. There was a flat wooden railing behind me, so I could sit up and hold court at 1 Prospect Krovatyu, as I thought 1 Bed Avenue would sound in Russian. I looked up at the clear dots in the pristine Siberian nighttime sky. Of all the places I had traveled in the world, nowhere had the stars seemed so vividly white, or close to the earth's horizon.

As I stared at the familiar constellations that reduced the notion of Siberian otherness, I contemplated what lay ahead. Dr. Filonov had told D that he wanted to give me a couple of days to recover from the journey before we started the first medical fast. It looked like the midnight-blue sky was enveloping me. *I am in Siberia, sleeping outside in the mountains, and I am perfectly at ease.*

Pulling out my phone, I expelled an inadvertent coo when I discovered that I had a bar, just enough to send a WhatsApp message to my support group. I sent them a description of my rustic wooden sleeping platform, describing how I had set up my sleeping bag to see Cassiopeia from bed and how, below me, the brook burbled and sang. The vast distance shortened when I received a message back from Janet as fast as a shooting star. It concluded, "Dad and I feel like you are at the end of the world . . . if not, you must be able to see it from there. We keep you close in our hearts."

Bird songs and the brook's perpetual melody greeted me when I woke. My cheeks were dewy. A flicker of something I once knew waved in my chest: *a brand-new day is before me.* Reverberations on the worn wooden steps announced that someone was coming. Dr. Filonov appeared with his nurse, Nora, panting at his side. "доброе утро, мишель. Как твои дела?" he said, asking how I was doing.

"*Dobre utro, Dr. Filonov! Harasho spala. Ya golodayu sevodnya?*" I wished him a good morning back and assured him that I had slept well. Magically well, I would have added, had I known the word. He nodded, looking pleased, and then pointed to his watch and said, "*Desyet.*" I was to go for my first treatment at ten. *Will I begin dry fasting today? Will I be able to do it?* When I tried to ask about it, he waved and said, "*Pàtom*, later," and then disappeared up the steps with Nora.

I sat up to read from the slim volume of Rumi poems I had brought with me. The thirteenth-century mystical Persian poet's verses inspired me to write in my journal before my first treatments: "As I prepare to dry fast with Dr. Filonov, I keep hearing from Vitali what a battle it will be. I understand this. Rumi writes, 'There is an invisible strength within us; when it recognizes two opposing objects of desire, it grows stronger.'"[1] I thought that my will to live was stronger than any thirst my body could generate. "My desire—may it grow stronger—is to be strong, fearless, and radiant the way I was at seventeen." If I was going to heal, I decided that I might as well aim high.

Leaving my sleeping niche in place, I went to wash up under the orange plastic spigot, a luxury I wouldn't have once I started dry fasting. No water and no lotions were to touch my body during the time I fasted; otherwise, I'd be interrupting cellular incineration.

When I reached for my phone, I saw that I wasn't the only one impatient for the treatments to begin. "Dad wants to know precisely what the good doctor is doing to you. He needs to know what these treatments are."

"Like father, like daughter," I wanted to write back.

I was sitting on the wooden steps of the treatment *dacha* when Vitali summoned me in. Dr. Filonov was still dressed in the same Adidas sweatshirt and dark gray sweatpants. In photographs I had seen, he wore scrubs at clinics where he was a guest doctor in Moscow, but, here in Altai, dress codes seemed irrelevant.

Massage tables were set up around the room, as if Dr. Filonov was prepared to administer multiple treatments simultaneously in the open space. Each table was constructed from two wooden benches pushed together, covered with a thin futon, and clad in a faded floral sheet. A rough-hewn wooden table stood against the back wall, covered in an assortment of glass jars and a few standard medical tools that I recognized, like a stethoscope. Sunlight shone through the small windows.

Vitali gestured for me to lie down on the massage table closest to the door, and Dr. Filonov listened to my heart and murmured his approval. Dr. Filonov started to give me what Vitali described as a liver massage. As he would often do, Vitali sat next to me on a stool during my treatments, observing, translating, and sometimes, to my dismay, taking photographs.

Organ massages are not typical in the United States, but Vitali told me that "liver massages have been used in traditional Russian medicine for centuries. Your liver is highly toxic from the pharmaceutical drugs." He explained that the massages would be used to support it throughout the extreme detoxification process that dry fasting would activate. The liver massage was oddly soothing, and I realized no one had ever palpated my liver before. It seemed to alleviate tension in my abdominal area.

It was followed by cupping, which I knew to be an ancient Chinese—and apparently, Siberian—method for decongesting cells and draining the lymphatic system. Dr. Filonov dipped a wand into a jar filled with spirits, lit it with a lighter, deftly placed it in the empty glass jar for a moment, and adhered the glass jar to my liver area. The skin inside the jar got sucked up, which was painful. All the same, I

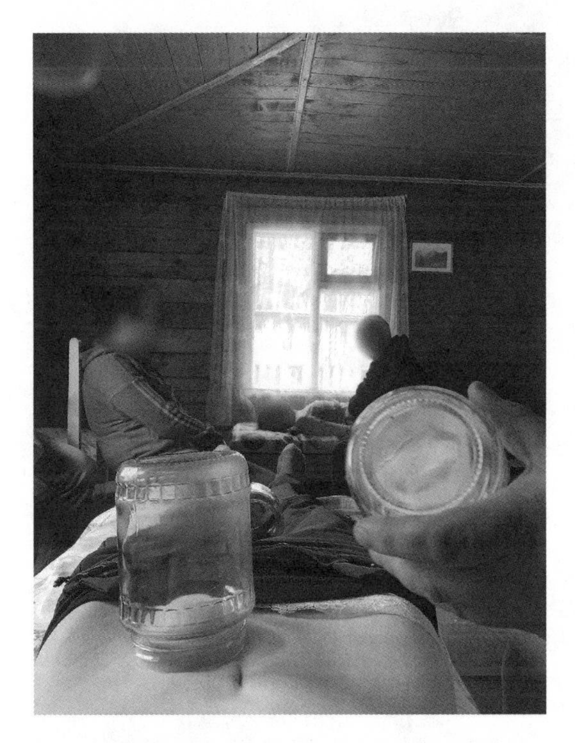

Cupping therapy in the treatment room

was determined not to show any discomfort during these treatments. I wanted to prove that I was a brave American patient who was prepared to go to any length to heal.

"*Terpimo?*" Dr. Filonov asked skeptically.

"He means, is it *tolerabile*?" Vitali piped up in Italiglish.

"*Ya silnaya*," I responded in Russian, meaning, "I am strong."

Then there was another stream of words that I didn't get, but Vitali translated. "It would be good for you to do some walking this afternoon, and then to do it every morning in the future when you dry fast." Dr. Filonov had already instructed Dmitri that I was to walk ten kilometers every day and that the distance between the center and the bridge to the main road was five kilometers. It didn't escape me that D had had to carry me to the car less than a week ago, but

I said with conviction that I would do it. I asked Vitali to translate that I was Dr. Filonov's most motivated patient. Dr. Filonov raised his eyebrows, and I realized this wasn't the first time he had heard such ambitious words.

8

STARVING IN SIBERIA WITH MY GULAG DOCTOR

The following afternoon, I experienced a surge of pain in my knees and joints from trying too hard to walk. I couldn't conceal my pain from Dr. Filonov, who decided that I would start dry fasting at once to reduce the inflammation. Dictated by pain, I rested the entire first day of dry fasting, without consciously thinking of what was to come. The gray sky mirrored my nebulous thoughts. But on the second day, I managed to walk five kilometers at a slow tempo to the bridge that overlooked the Ust-Sema river. Plunked down on a raised beam at the edge of the bridge, I peered into the eddying water, hoping its energy would rub off on me. Determination fueled my legs; I willed myself to walk in spite of being in a broken body.

At the bridge, I tapped out a message to my family: "You have never had a massage until you have been to Siberia. Dr. Filonov said my muscles were like stones and asked if I had ever had a massage. I said, 'All the time,' and he couldn't believe it. His massage is like the gulag, but it's effective."

Dry fasting this third time, when my body was so clean, was not as hard as the three-day fast had been at home; my body seemed to be adapting to this eccentric system of healing. I felt more contemplative and observant. On my walk back to the center, I admired the tall pines that lined the road, and the many ferns, emerald and sage, that grew at their feet. I took a photo to send home. I thought that if I created a visual proximity for Dad and Janet, they would be able to fill in the rest of the scene with their imaginations.

By the end of the day, when I was settled back down in my open-air camp on the landing, Janet, a fellow northern New Englander who relished her own walks in the woods, wrote, "I envy you the quiet space you have there in such an unspoiled setting . . . that in itself is great therapy." The photo journal was working; they were there with me in spirit.

Before I drifted off to sleep under the Siberian night sky, I wrote, "I just feel peaceful. My mouth is slightly dry. My spine hurts. I don't have a headache, but my knees are hurting. I feel fearless." Every day was a step into the profound unknown, and I yielded to it.

. . .

Dr. Filonov's two daughters arrived just as I started dry fasting. They had been working as therapists for their father during the summer sessions at the clinic for years. His youngest daughter, Anastasia, nicknamed Nastia, looked like a younger version of him, with the same dignified nose and bluish gray Slavic eyes. She wore her long blond hair in a high ponytail, off from her fair skin, and spoke a pleasant and passable form of English. She was training to be a nurse at the medical institute in Barnaul, with her husband, Dima, who was also a therapist for Dr. Filonov.

His eldest daughter, Olga, exuded an air of responsibility and duty, and her resemblance to her mother, Valentina, was remarkable. She took on many extra responsibilities at the center, I'd observe.

Nastia started administering my treatments as soon as she arrived, and we developed a friendly rapport. "Tell me about your father," she said that first day, her manner kind and inviting. Then she responded in turn when I asked, "Tell me about your daughter," who was staying with her paternal grandparents in Barnaul. Nastia's warm demeanor was characteristic of a good nurse; I felt nurtured by her.

The following morning, after a particularly aggressive treatment, I found another spot to sit along the Katun, the river that ran parallel to the dirt road. The new spot was about two thirds of the way to the bridge. I knew that the river's waters flowed all the way from a revered Siberian glacier located almost five hundred kilometers away, and that its temperature never rose above 55 degrees, even in summer. It was wider than some lakes I had seen, and I wouldn't want to fall in, for it was famed for whitewater rafting. It originated on Mt. Belukha, at 14,770 feet. It was the defining feature of Altai as far as I was concerned, and I learned later that it was the most famous river in all of Russia. Listening to the Katun roar with vitality was another form of healing therapy. If I had any anxiety or thought that I was obsessing about, I just mentally tossed it into the river's current and felt free. I had much to cast into the river that morning.

Nastia had inserted needles in the tensest muscles in my back to decongest them, and I wanted to cry because it was so excruciating, though I didn't. Then Dr. Filonov sent me off to walk ten kilometers. "Gulag," I called out jokingly as I walked out of the center. We had

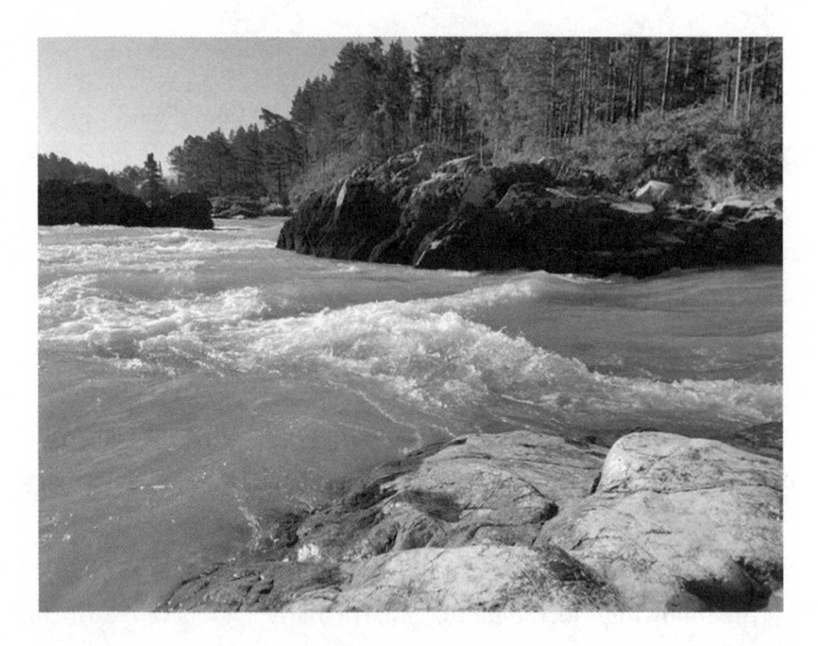

The mighty Katun river

developed a banter around exchanges like this. I kept calling Dr. Filonov the gulag doctor: "*Moy dorogoy vratch gulag!*" He would laugh. I could speak to him through the conduit of my broken Russian, Nastia's intermediate English, and Vitali's broken Franglish.

Once I was safely back to the center, I curled up in my outdoor perch to write to my family. "My mouth is getting dry, and I have five days left." I updated Janet and D on the strategy as I understood it: "I believe the plan is to dry fast for seven days, rehydrate for several days, and then dry fast for nine days. Dr. F thinks my body is too toxic to take nine straight days right away. He is monitoring my heart as we progress to make sure it is handling this well. The 'massages' are just what I imagine a torture chamber to be like."

Then I realized that my messages weren't going through, and I would have to resend them from the bridge in the morning. I turned to my journal instead, and I framed the period of dry fasting in comparison with the past months. "Five days of dry fasting for better health is an easy prospect when compared with the five months I just spent etiolated in bed."

• • •

Natasha brought her green summer-camp-style sleeping bag down to my perch to sleep outside with me. We could only communicate when we got a sliver of reception that enabled us to chat through Google Translate. Since there was no signal that night, we just made eye contact, smiled, put our hands on our hearts to signify empathy with one another's dry-fasting journey, and waved. The translations on our phones didn't always make sense, but from her messages and from the glint in her pale Russian-blue eyes, I could tell that she was fierce about healing.

In one of my messages, I asked why she was here, and she typed "mioma," without expounding on it, which I later figured out were uterine fibroids. In another bout of furious typing, she told me that she was on day six of a nine-day dry fast and that she didn't want to focus on the illness, but on the healing. "Be strong. We have to be strong, Michelle." This was Natasha's theme.

On my third morning of dry fasting, I woke up in surprise at how well I felt, so I reached to record it in my journal: "The thirst that plagued me on the first three-day dry fast is oddly absent, and my body seems to understand that we are in this for the long haul. I do feel weak this morning, and my tongue is dry, but it is certainly not intolerable. I wake with such peace that I could swear the river's mellifluous flow has healing properties. When I see the mist on the pines in the valley against the dark green mountains, I think of it as a morning gift." I settled into my routine of walking, treatments, and afternoon sunbathing with Rumi. I had no angst; I felt imbued with an aura of peace—one more profound than I had ever felt.

. . .

I awoke the next day missing my "Mr. Green Genes" smoothie from Juice Generation on Park Avenue and Twenty-Third. I could almost taste the thickness of the double-blended banana, kale, spinach, and hemp milk. I could hear myself saying, "Hold the mango; add almond butter." My thirst wasn't dire, but if I could have any wish, it would have been to swish that green smoothie through my teeth and around my mouth.

As the dry fasting progressed into day four, I seemed to be regaining my sense of humor. Every time Dr. Filonov came over to work on me in the treatment room, I cried out, "The gulag doctor is coming for me." That day he put a pillow under my head, and I said, "Ah, now it's a five-star gulag." Nastia found this hilarious, and she translated for me.

Dr. Filonov said solemnly, "You like to write books. You will write a book about 'Dry Fasting in the Siberian Gulag.'" Everybody was laughing. Dr. Filonov and I had established a good rapport. He said that my heart and body were tolerating the dry fasting very well. After a rigorous treatment on my legs, I took a much-deserved siesta by the river. I hadn't felt so carefree in a long time.

On the fifth morning, I awoke right after sunrise. I wrote in my journal, "I have a strong metallic taste in my mouth. My tongue is cracked, and it tastes like chemicals. My throat is sore. Dr. Filonov said last night that my liver is detoxing rapidly, as a result of the vast quantities of pharmaceutical drugs that I have consumed over the past six years."

Since I didn't have a mirror, I was obsessed with taking selfies of my tongue so I could examine it. By day five, it was encased in a thick, yellow, mucus-like paste that formed tiny ridges and patches across the entire surface. I shared a photo of my tongue with my

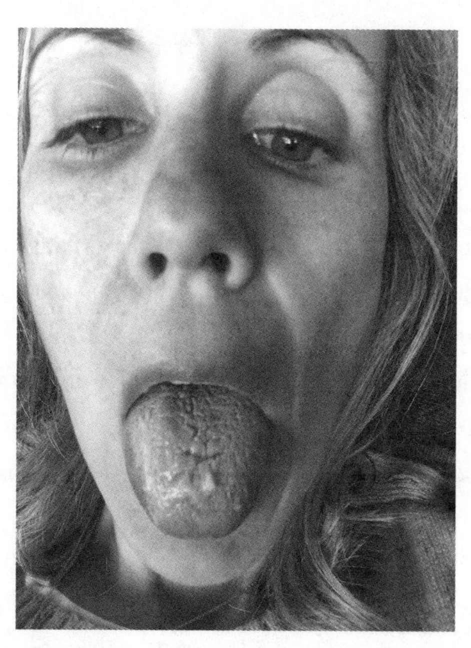

My tongue, during my nine-day dry fast at home in the Berkshires, November 2017

family, since it was the most apparent physical sign that I was dry fasting. "Quite a photo of your tongue," Janet wrote. She must have shuddered when she saw the picture.

I wanted to protect Dad and Janet from some of my ruminations, but in the middle of the seven-day dry fast, I wrote to D in a moment of despair. "I feel so dirty I could cry. My front teeth are caked with hardened mustard-yellow mucus. My hair. My body needs industrial cleaning." He fired back, "You are a real RGO now!" I could hear him laughing that I was in the former Soviet Union, his homeland, dirty and starving.

. . .

In hindsight, it was far easier to dry fast in Siberia than it had been alone at home. The supportive treatments alleviated my pain; being outside twenty-four hours a day meant that my mouth was far less dry. The walking routine, too, seemed to be integral to the fasting. Lena, Valentina, and Vitali were there with encouragement. Dr. Filonov, with Nastia at his side, observed and checked on me every day and evening. He kept telling me what a good job I was doing. I was in nature, away from the maddening fray of the world. All of this made it easier.

I had been squatting to pee outside, but as more staff arrived, I started using the wooden outhouses that had a hole in the ground to squat over. *I cannot be terribly dehydrated because I am still peeing at least seven times a day*. I hadn't expected this. I was also feeling increasingly better as the days progressed; my bodily sensation of heaviness and fatigue had been replaced with a sense of ease I hadn't known in years. The pain in my joints decreased, enabling me to walk more easily.

I scrawled some notes after my morning walk and treatments: "Very good treatment today. He said that I would have died if I had kept taking the antibiotics and fertility drugs. I could feel that. He said that the whole detox could take up to two years and that I have to keep dry fasting. He says I will return to full vitality."

Through Vitali and Nastia, I was gleaning fragments of the doctor's medical wisdom, which I shared with my family every day. "I just had a long conversation with Dr. Filonov about prescription pills, vitamins, and minerals. He said, 'Never take them. They are very bad for your liver.'" I made a vow that I wouldn't put any more crap in my body.

Dr. Filonov had waved his arms as he asked me, "Where do you think all of these prescription pills are going?" He gesticulated animatedly to my torso. "Straight through the liver, which filters everything. The liver is overburdened." I kept hearing him use a word that sounded like *hematologica*; it didn't take a linguist to understand that he was against the overuse of pharmaceutical drugs. In the past five years, I had taken thousands of prescription pills and vitamins, but I was now done with big pharma and all its subsidiaries.

When Dr. Filonov and Nastia did their rounds that night, they inspected my tongue again and shook their heads, for its state reflected the condition of my liver. They were kind about it, and encouraging, but all the same, after they left, my face wrinkled up to cry. I had worked so hard to be well the past five years, and it was rending to realize that all those efforts had actually led me backward, not forward. I crawled out of my sleeping bag to slip on my Birks and walk to the cheerful rivulet, hoping it would wash my sadness away.

Later that night, Vitali shot a short video of me while I was sitting up in my sleeping bag in my pale blue pajama shirt, sporting a very messy bun on top of my head.

"How are you feeling now?" Vitali asked.

"I just feel peaceful," I replied, adding, "thanks to the river's song."

"Do you have any symptoms tonight?" Vitali asked, while still shooting video footage.

"Nothing is really bothering me, other than that I had let big pharma get the best of me."

I was camera shy, though, and getting tired of feeling like I was being observed by everyone, all the time. So I asked Vitali if we could cut the camera to discuss Dr. Filonov's concerns about chemicals in our bodies, or *hematologica*, if I was hearing it right in Russian.

I was coming to see that the pharmaceutical industry didn't want to see me get well, because they wanted to keep peddling their drugs to me for years to come. The Food and Drug Administration is responsible for controlling the amounts of pesticide residue on our food, but that oversight clearly isn't working, because pesticides in food have been linked to the rampant rates of cancer and Alzheimer's in the United States. I told Vitali how my mom, an ardent environmentalist, used to read Rachel Carson's *Silent Spring* to me when I was a child. The book had been published in 1962—the warning sounded then about the dangers of pesticides. I went on, stating, "Dr. Filonov is right to be frustrated about the increased chemicals in the world that are making his patients so sick that they need to dry fast to get better."

This was a pet subject of Vitali's too, and we commiserated. Rachel Carson had posed a question that was perplexing us right there and then in Siberia, writing, "Future historians may well be amazed by our distorted sense of proportion. How could intelligent beings seek to control a few unwanted species by a method that contaminated the entire environment and brought the threat of disease and death even to their own kind? Yet this is precisely what we have done."[1]

Vitali said, "Michelle, how could we have done this to ourselves as a society? It's not just the poison in the medications and pesticides; it's in the air pollution and in the water. Dry fasting is a necessity in the twenty-first century, as Dr. Filonov says."

By now, though, my brain was getting tired; it didn't want to feel vexed while it fasted. I remembered the opening of an old Wendell Berry poem that I recited in fragments to Vitali, knowing he would appreciate it:

> A people in the throes of national prosperity, who
> breathe poisoned air, drink poisoned water, eat
> poisoned food,
> who take poisoned medications to heal them of the poisons
> that they breathe, drink, and eat[2]

He cried, "Michelle, that is exactly it! What is the name of that poem? When was it written? This is the reason we all should be dry fasting today!"

"It's 'The Reassurer,' and I think it was written in the sixties," I said. A haze had come over my brain, but it astonished me that I retrieved the Berry poem, an old skill I had lost long ago. I furrowed my brow and hung my head a little.

Vitali said, "I'm sorry, we should not be talking about upsetting things while you are dry fasting. I don't want to take away your positive energy. You are very tired, I see. We talk later."

After he departed, I wriggled around to get cozy in my nest of a sleeping bag, I let out a sigh so deep the sleeping platform seemed to vibrate with it. *On to day six*. I was adept at being my own cheerleader night and day. I went to sleep envisioning the vivacious Michelle that Dr. Filonov kept promising, free from the chemicals burdening my poor liver.

...

I woke up and unzipped myself from the sleeping bag to curve into a yogic half-moon pose under the cool morning sun. Now September, it was fleece-jacket temperature in the Siberian mornings, but it rose to a warm-your-bones temperature by early afternoon.

It was unfathomable to me that I could barely walk to the bathroom a week ago but that my adrenalin and sheer determination were fueling these quotidian walks. When I checked my phone that morning at the bridge, I found that Janet had written an encouraging note: "You are the toughest nut on the planet!" I felt as I were saying to Lyme disease, *I'm not going to let you vanquish my life*, and with that, I started up the dirt road back to the center and into day six, singing the days out loud, "One, two, three, four, five, six!" I added a slight lilt as I sounded out each day, rising to a crescendo that peaked at the "six."

...

The warm Siberian sun was healing me. After my treatment, I rested on top of my puffy yellow sleeping bag and felt the sunlight penetrating into my bones. I listened to the river's song while reading Rumi's poems: "One of the marvels of the world is the sight of a soul sitting in prison with the key in its hand."[3] Here I was, coming out of my Lyme prison and the key in my hand was Dr. Filonov's dry fast. As I read, I kept silently exclaiming, *But that's me! It's like it was written for me.*

When Dr. Filonov and Nastia asked how Natasha and I were feeling that night during their rounds, I reported, "I'm amazed at how much energy I have on day six. I have a metallic feeling in my mouth and esophagus, but my tongue doesn't feel too dry." They built me up with positive energy to carry me into day seven, and I smiled back while patting my heart in Miche sign language to show my appreciation.

Siberia! Sweet Siberia! had sent me encouraging messages, and I responded, "You have no idea how much these messages from you and D boost my morale."

My family's solidarity, coupled with Dr. Filonov's kindness, touched me. Tears from unidentified emotions moistened my dry cheeks, and I sought solace in tracing the seven sister stars of the Pleiades constellation. I could hear the echo of my mother's voice explaining that Atlas was the Greek titan holding up the sky, and the seven sisters were his daughters, conceived by the ocean goddess Pleione. To my childhood eyes, the seven seemingly tiny stars that formed this unique configuration had looked like the Eiffel Tower. Now I repeated their names to myself. Maia, Electra, Alcyone, Taygete, Asterope, Celaeno, and Merope. Then, I noticed how strange it was, how easily those names had come to me. *I wonder if my memory is coming back?* My sleep that night, so far into the fast, was intermittent.

On the seventh day, I woke up at dawn with an urgent need to pee, so I swiftly tucked my Kleenex packet into my pocket, slipped on my Birks, and, realizing I wouldn't make it to the outhouse, took off for the nearest patch of woods. I had my period, to my dismay. I was feeling weak, but after I went back to the *dacha* to fish a tampon out of the dark reaches of my suitcase, I took off on my ten-kilometer walk.

I was barely able to thrust one foot in front of the other, but I made it to the bridge and heaved myself onto the beam. I stared into the rippling river for a long time before I could stand again. I WhatsApped D about my period and faintness. Like a *babushka*, he said this worried him, and he warned me not to overdo it, saying to me, "Perhaps this is enough for the first time? See what the doctor says." I decided I'd apprise Dr. Filonov, and he would decide my course.

It took me almost three hours to make the round trip. When I was passing the open field on the left, the milestone that marked the final climb to the center was just ahead, my legs refused to go any farther. I sat down in the wildflowers by the side of the road and WhatsApped Dr. Filonov.

A few minutes later, Vitali and Lena showed up with the car, looking alarmed. "I'm okay, guys! I'm just spent." When Dr. Filonov examined me in the treatment room, he said, "You have finished this round." I was at peace with his decision, knowing I had given every atom of effort I had.

He continued, saying it had been "an excellent first effort" but that the menstruation had initiated a different kind of cleansing.

I was scared that I wouldn't make it through the next critical nine-day fast, and I communicated my fear through Nastia. "Don't worry," she translated back in her calming tone. "Everything will be okay. On the second attempt at fasting, you will accomplish nine days." I nodded, reassured.

After Nastia gave me a soothing abdominal massage, they sent me to bed in the *dacha*. I wasn't to sleep outside the next few days because the immune system is very vulnerable immediately following a dry fast, and I was told that it must be protected. I was instructed to rest.

As soon as I was tucked into bed, Valentina appeared at my bedside. She was holding my purple thermos, filled with hot water, and bubbling away in a rapid Russian that I couldn't understand at all. I smiled feebly at her and said, "*Spasibo*." She poured hot water into a glass cup and handed it to me.

I curled my hands around the cup and raised it to my eager mouth. When the hot water hit my tongue, I let it sink deep into the ridges. It tasted sweet, as if it had honey in it, although it did not. With each hydrating sip, I felt like a wilted plant whose blossoms were perking up upon being watered. I closed my eyes to take stock of my situation.

I had made it. Round one.

I had gone without food or water for seven days, and I was alive and well. As my entire body relaxed with that knowledge, I realized how much tension I'd been holding in order to make this rigorous effort. But now it was time to rest.

I had been asleep for two hours when Dr. Filonov checked on me. "Keep sleeping; it's very good that you have no nausea," he said through Nastia. My ears had started ringing when I first drank water, but he said that was normal. *Rest it is, dear body*, I told myself. I drifted back into a sleep more profound than I had known in years—and without the dreaded Ambien.

9

THE BODY IS THE DOCTOR

When I woke to another dose of my precious elixir of hot Siberian spring water, I sat up and took a selfie of myself looking bright and radiant, sipping from my cup of hot water. I sent it to D and Janet with the caption, "I survived 7 days no food no water." I typed out the words, "Thank you for all of the support. It would be immeasurably harder for me without the three of you. It's time to carefully rehydrate me."

Janet fired off a text right away, in the middle of their night, so I know that they must have been keeping their ringer on in the final days of this first extended dry fast. "Wow, what a survivor you are! Hoping you are feeling at least a wee bit better by now."

That morning, Lena brought me a thermos and said, "*Kompot!*" I had to write and ask D what compote was, and he explained that it was juice made from boiling fruits like apples, pears, raisins, and apricots. I skeptically poured some of the dark plum-colored viscous liquid into my cup. It was so cloying that I could barely swallow it,

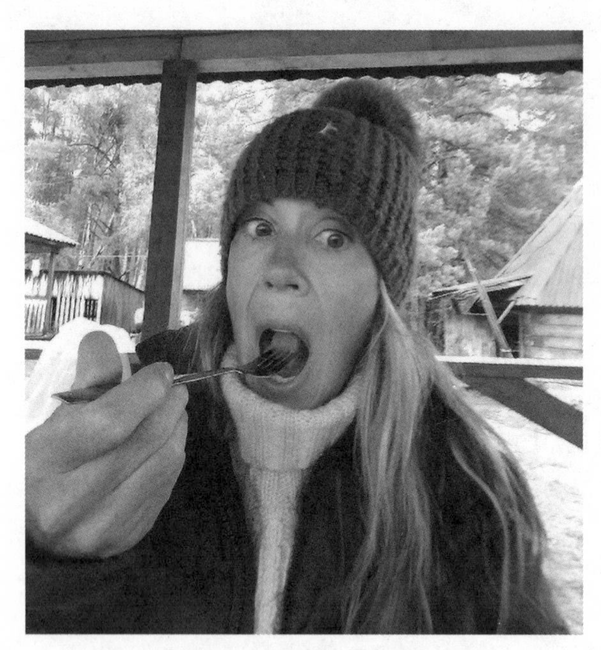

First watermelon on the exit

even though no sugar had been added. When Nastia and Dr. Filonov made their rounds later, I held the compote up and grimaced. They quickly exchanged a few words and Nastia said, "You need glucose for your brain, so if you don't like the compote, you will have *arbuz* now."

"Watermelon?"

"Yes. Father says it is very good for the kidneys."

I padded over to the outdoor picnic table to feast on juicy watermelon for breakfast. My body perked up with every bite of succulent fruit, and Nastia announced that I would have kasha and salad later on.

Now that I'd survived, and the worry had subsided on both sides of the Atlantic, D started joking over WhatsApp. "If Michelle stays on the Russian program when she gets back, our food budget will be chopped by two thirds. Russian kasha and cabbage are cheap! Works for me!" The levity was short-lived for me, for I knew that the journey ahead was daunting. I didn't know anyone who had survived nine days with no food and no water. Yet Dr. Filonov had successfully guided hundreds of patients through nine-day dry fasts, and I trusted him.

I continued to rest over the next few days because I felt increasingly dizzy, tired, and weak. Dr. Filonov assured me that these were normal symptoms after dry fasting, and that I shouldn't overanalyze them. "You need to gather your forces for the next big dry fast," he said. Between naps, I reported to the treatment room for a type of full-body decongestive massage that is only conducted at the center after a patient has exited a dry fast. During it, honey is applied to different regions of the body and then tapped until it turns into a paste. The tapping becomes vigorous until the skin, covered in the tacky honey paste, is lifted up and down, painfully. The process feels brutish and is quite the opposite of a relaxing Swedish massage.

After a couple of days in the cabin, I went back down to my sleeping bag outside. In spite of the beaming light of the nearly full moon, I enjoyed the deepest sleep that I can ever remember. Each morning, I'd wake with the sensation that warm molasses was running through my veins, nearly weeping in gratitude for the peace and the respite from pain that I felt.

When I opened my eyes one morning, I saw that someone had put a thermos of hot water with dried apricots next to my sleeping bag. This was the work of Vitali. He frequently spoke in admiration of the Hunza tribe in Pakistan that primarily consumed apricots, whose people lived to be 120 years old. I sat up to witness the sun's rose-colored hues against the dark Siberian fir-covered mountains and sipped the delicious nectar with gratitude. My body was not in pain—a respite that had seemed impossible to fathom just a month before. The intense joint pain in my knees and back had abated. I felt like I was shining inside, filled with the same rosiness as the sun.

• • •

As I exited from the dry fast, I turned philosophical. I considered how dry fasting had enabled my body to draw on its natural healing abilities. Thoughts about rediscovering my faculty of intuition were dancing in my head. I reached for my journal and scrawled rapidly before I forgot the interesting words coming to me: "The body is the doctor."

I was breathing through my nose perfectly for the first time in years. My sinuses had never been so clear in my entire life. My sinuses didn't even clog up at night, or in the dusty cabin. Between my lifelong allergy to dust, my intolerances to dairy and gluten, the mold exposure, and perhaps other unidentified factors, I always had been the girl with the plugged-up nose who had to breathe through her mouth. Now, as I sat, I could smell the delicate apricots and the Christmas scent of the handsome Siberian firs. Beforehand, I could have nestled in a garbage dump and smelled nothing. *Smelling is a miracle. I can't enumerate all these miracles.*

When I took my first *bania* bath in eight days and inspected my body, I gasped when I saw that the skin on my elbows and arms was like brand new. When I'd arrived, my arms had been covered in the silvery scales and raised red bumps of psoriasis. These were gone. I ran my hands up and down my arms and over the back sides of my elbows to make sure, but there was nothing there but soft skin. I massaged hydrating coconut oil over my body, then sat in the *bania* and wept in surreal disbelief. As I washed, I played Beethoven's "Ode to Joy" from the Ninth Symphony in my mind.

I had begun to think of it as marathon training. I was training my body to increase its endurance for dry fasting, similar to how a runner trains for a marathon. Dry fasting was starting to reap benefits, and I had worked up to this next level of training.

A voice from the primordial depths of my brain wondered if I would ever feel fully rejuvenated. While much of my body felt better, the palms of my hands and the soles of my feet still hurt. As I had recovered and rehydrated, the tinnitus in my ears returned. *Would the nine-day dry fast cure it?* I had felt groggy ever since exiting the dry fast, so I didn't know if the debilitating chronic fatigue had been healed. These pesky doubts crowded my head until, eventually, I had to be stern with myself. I had no alternative but to see whether dry fasting for nine days would kill me or cure me. The worries were the result of being chronically ill and a prisoner of my symptoms for so long.

10

EXITING TO REENTER

> But the day when I rose at dawn from the bed of perfect
> health, refresh'd, singing, inhaling the ripe breath
> of autumn, . . . O then I was happy.
>
> —**Walt Whitman,** "When I Heard at the Close of the Day"

What dumbfounded me was that I felt weaker in the days that followed than I had during the dry fast itself. Dr. Filonov reiterated that this was normal, but I naïvely thought I would feel rejuvenated as soon as I started sipping the prized hot water. Even though I believed that dry fasting would save me, I was worried that I remained so weak. Weakness had been a constant for years.

I didn't want to alarm Dad and Janet, so I sent my worries separately to D. On WhatsApp, D asked Dr. Filonov directly about my weakness, and Dr. Filonov patiently repeated the same message he had told me: "Michelle's body was so toxic from the antibiotic treatments and Lyme that the effects of dry fasting are more dramatic in her. The cleansing accelerates when we start drinking water. It doesn't end with dry fasting." In other words, the dry fasting triggered a landslide of bacterial debris, and the influx of hot water called forth an invisible multi-fleet garbage truck service that was now moving around my body to clear it all out.

Dr. Filonov also explained that the fast was generating a new immune system as it killed off damaged white blood cells and created new white blood cells. The fast triggered my body to grow new stem cells, too. I tried to imagine how hard my body was working to heal me on the inside. I saw armies of cells carrying out sophisticated tasks that were intangible to me.

I slept like a hibernating bear during the entire week. When I wasn't sleeping, I was eating Lena's healing meals. I looked at Lena with pleading eyes when she set an enormous portion of oatmeal in front of me. I pushed it away and tried to show how big it looked to me with widespread hands: "*Bolshoi*, Lena, *Bolshoi*!" I wanted to ask for a Lilliputian-sized portion, but that far transcended my linguistic capacities. We settled on wee bowls of the pretty yellow grains with finely diced apricots; it sounded like "*pesheno*" to me when they said it in Russian. After not eating for over a week, the nutty taste of the millet mixed in with the sweet apricot spread deliciousness from my mouth to my stomach. I rested in between meals, listening to Handel's *Messiah* or Bach's cello suites through my headphones.

The outside world was a faraway place, about which I knew little, and it faded for me as I focused on recovering from Lyme disease. I had no idea that Hurricane Harvey was taking place in Houston, because D wanted to protect me from this devastating news. I would only learn of this natural disaster and its effects much later.

Natasha was well into her exit at this point, and she called me her "little sister" in WhatsApp messages. I wasn't sure why she was so protective of me, but when she broke her fast and had more energy to write, she sent me a long message that I pasted into the Google Translate app.

As Natasha recounted, when Dmitri and Valentina picked her up from the airport, D had said, "My wife is very ill, and I'm worried about her. She needs support and strength. Please look after her if you can." She thought his care for me was so poignant that she started to love me like a little sister even before we met. I realized a deep friendship was taking root there in Siberia, one that was not contingent on language.

Each time I saw Natasha, she flashed her strong blue eyes at me as if she was on fire with lightning bolts of joy. I asked Dr. Filonov why Natasha had dry fasted for nine days and looked like she could climb a mountain, whereas I could barely stand up. "Do not compare yourself to her," he told me sternly through Nastia. "She was not nearly as sick as you are. Do not compare yourself with any of the other patients right now."

More patients had started to arrive, coming from all parts of Russia. Soon there were nearly thirty of us, and the center began to resemble a village scene in a Brueghel painting. I observed a confident woman about my age, clad in a traditional flax dress, carry a tent to the field facing the gate, where she set it up. A tall woman with short red hair entered my *dacha* and claimed the twin cot near mine. I gleaned from my broken Russian that she was from the Siberian city of Novosibirsk. A petite blond lady from Irkutsk set up camp on the cot by the door, nodding her head at me with a diffident smile.

A few patients were eager to meet the American who had come from New York. Some spoke a smattering of English, but they were saving their energy for the extended dry fasting. Most were there to dry fast between nine and eleven days. It is taxing on the brain to search for words in another language while the brain is not being fed. Most of the patients just gawked at me in silence. I wrote to my family, "It's humorous to me that so many Russians have paid to starve in Siberia."

"That irony has not eluded us," Janet replied. I knew that message had been worded by Dad, who didn't use a cell phone of his own; he had found his sense of humor about this, too.

They all called my doctor Sergey Ivanovich, out of respect and affection, so I began to do the same. No one else called him Dr. Filonov, and I wanted to be a chameleon as much as the only American in Siberia could.

The unspoken code was that one didn't speak about one's illness; we were merely dry fasting together in solidarity. I learned from Nastia that there were patients with cancer, rheumatoid arthritis, the complications of old age, fertility issues, and some who just wanted to lose weight.

The rest of Dr. Filonov's staff had arrived. Dr. Filonov's nephew Andrei had the responsibility of driving the bus full of patients from the Barnaul airport to the center, but he was also an advanced therapist. Andrei stood tall at over six feet with a belly that surely had Siberian bear DNA in it. Dr. Filonov had been training Andrei for years, and Andrei was an expert at liver manipulations, deep cellular massages, cupping, and other treatments. Andrei also excelled at making inappropriate jokes, although I was mostly spared from these since I didn't understand them.

Andrei would ask if I wanted *shashliki*, otherwise known as Russian barbecue, while I was dry fasting. "What do you think about American politics and Putin, Michelle?" My linguistic shortcomings saved me from answering. When we took excursions in his old Mercedes minibus and encountered cows crossing the road, he would say in English,

"Fresh meat," and pretend to run into them while we squealed, aghast. Andrei could not be serious unless he was treating a patient.

As other patients came to populate the benches in the treatment room, I was surprised that the therapists spoke animatedly to one another and to the patients during treatments. They would pause while giving treatments to answer their loud cell phones. The patients chattered with one another as they lay on tables half undressed, so it felt like the quiet room had become a kind of bazaar.

I appreciated the way Dr. Filonov structured the days for the patients who had come for a three-week dry-fasting program. They arrived typically on day two of their fast, and they had treatments between mid-morning and mid-afternoon. There were various excursions in the afternoon, which helped divert the patients' minds from thoughts of food and water. In the evenings, around the fire pit, Dr. Filonov gave extended lectures on dry fasting. It was as if Socrates had appeared; all his patients gathered around him, listening with rapt expressions on their faces. I watched his eyes in the light of the fire as he patiently explained the science of dry fasting and answered questions at length long into the night.

When I pestered Nastia about his lectures, she told me that her father shared medical facts, anecdotes, and tips on how to adopt healthy practices at home. Sometimes he would share a patient testimonial. "Michelle, you know he can talk endlessly on the kidneys or the liver and all sorts of medical things." Although Dr. Filonov was frequently laconic, and his text messages were always succinct, he could lecture for hours about his passion for the science of dry fasting. He was the world expert on this subject, and that was why we were all there, even though the world knew of him only mythically, through a single quotation that circulates on the internet in somewhat obscure circles.

On my morning walks, for the first time, I was not alone. There were strangers from other cabins walking up and down the road, men and women of all ages dressed in various layers of motley clothing and rubber boots. I heard a few curt "*Dobre utros*"—the customary morning greeting—but some just ignored me and kept walking. A rotund man in an expensive Arc'teryx jacket—an odd sight in Siberia—muttered, "Good morning" to me, and I realized this must be the husband of the woman with the MSR tent that had popped up in the field; they were conspicuously gear savvy.

I could see that the constant questions and the careful monitoring that the doctor offered his patients took a toll. In the early mornings, I frequently saw him walking in the woods with Nora and disappearing near the river. One day I walked home on that path, and I saw evidence of a campfire, which I surmised to be his own retreat. His work was grave and serious, and he needed a respite.

As the days passed, I built anticipation for my next, potentially life-changing dry fast. Each morning I walked, chatted over breakfast with Natasha via our fallible Google Translate, and underwent a treatment. I tried to integrate myself into the larger group of patients, although I felt overwhelmed and shy given my linguistic limitations, whereas I had felt more confident when I was nearly the only patient on site.

A woman about my age from St. Petersburg, wearing a traditional Russian linen dress, approached me one day. She had a long braid down her back. I recognized her as the one with the MSR tent. "Hello, Michelle. I am Tania. Sergey Ivanovich sent me to translate for you if you need help." Her English was impeccable and, though she was dry fasting, we managed to have conversations as long as she was able. She had come from St. Petersburg to fast with her husband, in order to improve their fertility. Days later, after she broke her fast, she collected *kalina* berries and made a jar of red *kalina* marmalade for me, with a label on it that read, "Kalina for gentle Michelle." Tania had to conserve her voice as well, but I knew we'd have been kindred spirit friends if there had been more time.

. . .

When Dr. Filonov encouraged me to go on excursions, he asked Natasha to look after me. Riding in the car with Yuri, one of the massage therapists, she sang along to old Russian songs while I suffered each bump as the car flew over the dirt roads. She didn't notice the bumps, but they drained my feeble energy. We stopped at some caves near the famous Denisova cave where archeologists had found the 41,000-year-old bones of a juvenile girl. When I saw that we had to hike up to the caves, I blanched. Natasha bounded up the narrow paths while I tottered up them, clinging to tree branches as I went. When she reached the top, I looked high above me and saw her cry out, "*Ya silnaya!*" She pumped her fists and jumped up and down, whereas I sat right down on the trail to wait for her as she explored the caves.

When we got back to the center, I nearly passed out again and ended up sleeping the entire next day. Dr. Filonov wasn't pleased. "You were supposed to look up at the caves, not hike. We are rebuilding your immune system. It is critical that you rest. Hiking is for later." I hadn't understood, and I apologized for jeopardizing my healing process. We both looked frustrated, our communication stalled without a skilled translator to smooth things.

Afterward, as I reflected on the incident, I wrote in my journal, "I overdid it yesterday when I was already down. I didn't sleep the full moon night, and I was weak that day. I must voice my needs. For example, 'No, I can't go. No, I need to rest.' Although my will can override messages from my body warning me to be cautious, I cannot keep depleting my fragile energetic reserves."

After a few days of rest, we were to go on another excursion, and I could tell that it was a special one from the excited look on Natasha's face. We had only sunny days in Siberia, and this was no exception. We walked over a red pedestrian suspension bridge with tourists and families to cross the mighty Katun river. The path took us through the woods for a couple of kilometers on a gentle rolling incline until we came to a cascading waterfall, and it finally dawned on me that *vodapad*, a word I'd been hearing, meant waterfall. We stripped down to our bathing suits to frolic under the falling water. Natasha relished the cold water and cried out in joy, but I didn't have the strength to linger. We sat on rocks to dry out, and gesticulated to one another, since language wasn't possible. I didn't understand that we would be taking a boat back to the starting point, but she escorted me down another path to a boat launch. There was a motorized raft waiting for us, and Natasha shrieked with joy as we sped off down the Katun. The rapid movement made me feel like throwing up, and I could imagine hearing Dr. Filonov's stern admonition to be gentle.

Natasha's face was still radiant as a child's when we returned to the center, but I was limping along, exuding fatigue. Dr. Filonov looked at me and shook his head in exasperation. "We are doing leeches tonight," Nastia called out when I tried to skirt them and make my way to my sleeping bag. 1 Bed Avenue, Siberia, would have to wait.

"This will cleanse your blood. It's very good for you," Nastia said as I followed her into the treatment room. I brought my eye pillow from the airplane and headphones, because I didn't want to see or hear anything about these leeches. I listened to Chopin nocturnes as leeches sucked my blood. The mild sensation that I was being eaten produced a grimace on my face. "It's okay, Michelle. Don't worry," Nastia reassured me. After she removed the leeches, she taped pads to my liver to catch the blood that would be leaking out overnight. It made me want to escape my body for a few hours. I fled the torture chamber to take refuge in the billowing folds of down in my cozy nest.

I had begun to think of Monday, September 11, as the day to start the big *golodanye*, as dry fasting is called in Russian (literally "starvation"). Although I didn't share it with anyone, I thought it would be symbolic to start dry fasting on the most tragic day in my country's history, as if I were dry fasting in honor of those who had lost their lives September 11, 2001. I had a murky theme of death and rebirth in my mind, but I wasn't intellectually alert enough to articulate it.

In keeping with the symbolism of September 11, and since I had seen some patients conduct eleven-day dry fasts, I started having aspirations to dry fast for eleven days rather than nine. I thought that if nine days were critical, eleven might be even more healing and cleansing for my body. When I mentioned this to Dr. Filonov, he said, "*Posmotrim.*" I had learned that this, his favorite expression, meant "We will see."

Over the weekend, we had an excursion planned to a sacred cedar forest frequented by shamans, on the Mongolian border. Dr. Filonov's eyes lit up when he said that I should go. "It will give you energy for the nine-day dry fast."

Natasha and I boarded the bus together. From the window I could see gentle green-nubbed mountains. As the ride continued, the mountains grew jagged, white-capped. I felt Natasha's shoulder warm next to mine, even as the air chilled as we ascended. I knew we were in the land of the shamans when I saw the vast cedar forest in the distance decorated with prayer flags. I meandered alone through the cedars, accompanied by my thoughts on these sacred Altai spaces.

The remaining indigenous Altai people and their shamans still revere their sacred mountains, rivers, and spirits. I had read that each *seok*, or clan, has a sacred mountain called *yiyk tuu*. Each valley, each mountain peak, and each spring has its own spirits that are called *eezi*. I felt a kinship with the Altai people, for I, too, regarded the mountains and rivers as contributing to my healing. I felt a deep respect for this cedar forest.

One ancient cedar beckoned to me with white prayer flags hanging from its outstretched arms; offerings of coins and trinkets had been placed around its roots. I sat down and leaned against the dark orange and cream bark of its sprawling trunk to contemplate the task ahead. Each time I thought of starting to fast again, my heart quickened, betraying a nervousness I didn't want to acknowledge. I wanted to be stoic, but when I sat under the cedar and looked out over the Mongolian steppe, I realized that I felt slightly skittish. I inhaled a long breath at largo tempo and exhaled the tension in my chest and shoulders. I kept breathing until the calm that only meditation can generate settled into me.

I had seen a lively Mongolian market from the bus, so I wandered back to where we had been dropped off. Dozens of booths were set up alongside the highway. People had come out of the Siberian woods to barter. There were patterned socks, knit out of yak wool, selling for about five dollars. Soft cream cashmere hats were selling for 3,500 rubles, or about fifty dollars, but I hadn't brought enough rubles with me to buy souvenirs that day. Natasha found me and told me through Tania that Dr. Filonov wanted me to buy certain herbs to take home and steep into tea. She helped me pick them out, and I bought a small bag of creamy-looking Siberian pine nuts for D, since they were being sold by the kilo at a fraction of their price in the United States.

When we returned to the center that afternoon, I gathered my toiletries and strode to the *bania*. By my estimate, this would be my last bath for eleven days. I scrubbed every square centimeter of my body before I emerged in my freshly laundered blue pajamas.

As I stepped out of the *bania* rosy and clean, Dr. Filonov came over with Vitali. He took a firm stance on the ground. I recognized this posture from when he'd look at his patients during the lectures by the fire pit. "You are strong enough to do this in spite of your weak body. You have the spirit of the Siberian Altai mountains."

He paused as I considered what I had learned about Altai, which is described in Buddhist texts as a portal connecting the earth with spiritual realms. Perhaps this is why the ancient practice of shamanism thrives in this part of the world. All nature in the Siberian Altaian perspective is animate, from each rivulet to each mountain crevice. Buddhists thought that the revered Mount Belukha, a few hundred kilometers from the center, was the site of *Shambhala*, a pure spiritual land on earth. If I had the spirit of the Siberian Altai mountains, that was a high honor.

My Siberian doctor was not a loquacious man, so I listened, attentive, as Vitali attempted to translate. "I know that meditation is important to you, and there is a site by the Katun river that is very strong for meditation. It is at the confluence of three rivers. I will drive you there tomorrow. It is meant for someone who is close to spirit." Meditation is also venerated in Altai, and Dr. Filonov appreciated that I was a lifelong meditator.

He turned his dignified profile to the mountains in the distance, as if he were deciding whether to continue. "When I told my Russian-born American patients that you were coming, they thought an American would struggle with this treatment and this place, but what they didn't know is that you have a rare and strong soul. You were meant to come here." His voice rose in a crescendo as he concluded, proclaiming, "You are like the native ones from Altai. You will go home and shine and write your books!"

I walked away trembling in a mélange of hopeful disbelief at the thought of shining. If my body was a temple, it had decayed over the past years to the point of being near condemned, but this doctor gave me hope that it could be renovated. The results of the seven-day fast had showed me it was possible. Dr. Filonov said that my body was lagging behind my mind and my will, or spirit. *Can it catch up? He says that I will be able to write again. Could I really come back to life? I believe him.* After the seven-day dry fast started to clear out the Lyme cobwebs in my brain, I thought, *Have I been hiding behind Lyme disease?* I never thought my brain would work properly again. Having lost my purpose as a professor and writer, I had checked out of life. Dr. Filonov's uplifting pep talk made me want to come out of hiding from the shadows of my illness.

Since we weren't allowed to have dinner the night before a dry fast, I spent my last evening sipping water that poured right out of the mossy Siberian mountain into my purple metal thermos. I couldn't take those last sips for granted, for they'd have to last for eleven days.

I wanted to set an intention on this symbolic evening in the most magical place I knew. I walked down the dirt road, lined by sky-high Siberian pine trees interspersed with gleaming white birch trees, until I reached the clearing where the glacial Katun billows down from the sacred mountain of the Buddhist *Shambhala* legends, Belukha. *If you heal, perhaps you can climb Belukha one day.* I sat on a gray rock the size of a chaise longue, as close to the fierce azure water as I could get. The Katun seduced me, for I had stagnated for so long. "Flow," it said. "Just flow. No stagnation, no fear. Let go and flow!"

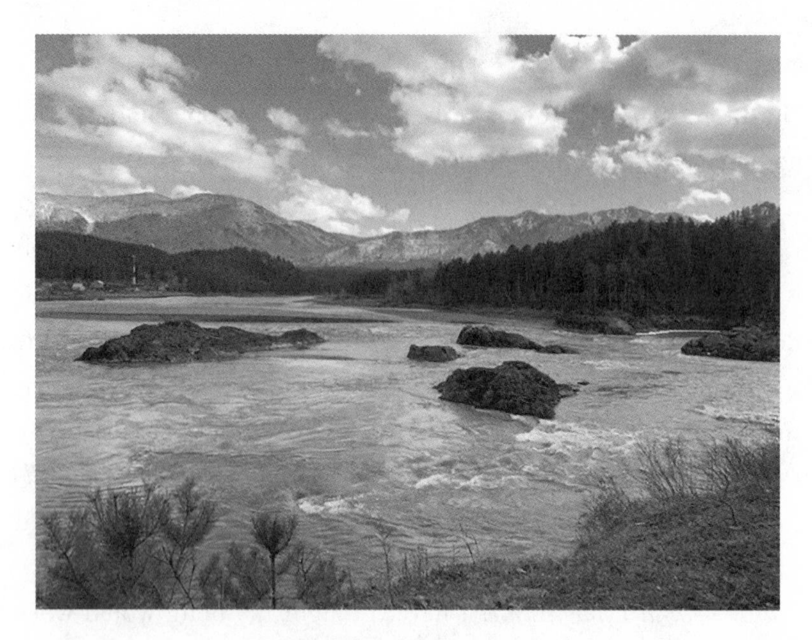

My meditation site at the Katun river

Under the warmth of the Altai sun, I pulled my worn journal out of my pocket to set an intention:

> This is a rebirthing we are witnessing. As I prepare to dry fast for nine to eleven days with Dr. Filonov, I know that this is a fight, a fight to get my life back. I am stronger than these diseased cells and spirochetes. If this radical treatment of starving myself in Siberia works, I vow to share it with others who might be close to burning out their wicks, too. My intention, as I set it here, and cast it into the Katun, is to be vibrant, and produce meaningful work that I can share as a testament to the resiliency of the human body. I have told my mind, body, and spirit what their upcoming jobs are: my body is the doctor, my mind rests, and my spirit holds space for the body to work.
>
> *Ya gotava*, I am ready.

I may have been the most eager person in history to starve, as I prepared for the most important segment of my medical journey to fight Lyme. I walked back to the center with purpose in my step.

11

MY NINE-DAY DRY FAST UNDER THE SIBERIAN SUN

Fasting is the greatest remedy. It's the physician within.

—Attributed to Philippus Paracelsus

Over the preceding days, a few people had brought their sleeping bags down to the landing by the dam, and they often wandered around at night talking. So I'd returned to the porch of the *dacha*. I lay there and tried to sleep. The women inside, who were in their nine-day dry fasts, were having trouble sleeping, and they chattered together. In my sleeping bag on the porch, I fretted. It was impossible to sleep and, without sleep, I wouldn't be able to endure this dry fast. I woke before my alarm sounded, frustrated by this inauspicious start. I had slept so well fasting before the throng of patients arrived. *Would I be able to sleep in the midst of the fray with thirty patients on site?*

Natasha was leaving that morning, and I didn't want to miss our farewell. She was about to climb into the car when I found her. Her face radiated light, and she told me in English, "I love you, little sister." I hugged her and waved until the car drove her out of my sight. I was on my own to embark on the grand *golodanye*.

Since the ten-kilometer walk was the most daunting task of the day while dry fasting, and since it was my only responsibility, I liked to set off at once upon waking. Then, as soon as my treatments were finished, I had the remainder of the day to rest and read as I pleased. I had already memorized this walk. The tall pines whispered in the breeze to me with the bass continuo of the Katun in the offing. Songbirds landed on wildflowers. It felt like nature was supporting my healing journey. One of the other patients told me that less than 3 percent of Russia was protected as a nature reserve, but the revered Altai mountains were an exception, for at least 20 percent of the land had been protected. The United Nations Educational, Scientific and Cultural Organization (UNESCO) had also made efforts to conserve land in Altai.

My mind wandered as I walked. Valentina had confided in Dmitri that Dr. Filonov was very "democratic," as she put it, which meant that he wanted the center's treatments to be accessible to everyone. He kept the program costs very low. I admired his altruism and the sacrifices that his family made to treat patients in the Altai mountains. He had outhouses and a communal treatment room, not a steel-and-glass clinic cantilevered over a hillside like some I had seen in western Europe, where patients still looked fatigued and sick after years of expensive treatments and thousands of euros spent on pills.

Dr. Filonov drove a rugged old Soviet SUV called a Neva. He had the heart of a healer who wasn't looking to keep patients coming back to him for years. He was looking to heal patients once and for

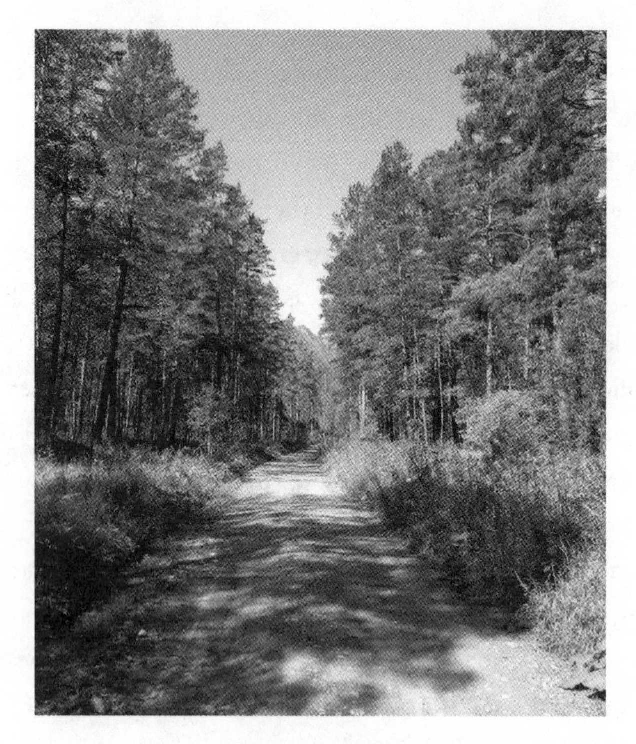

The walking road

all, for a meager fee of fifty dollars a day, which included unlimited access to him on WhatsApp, treatments, lodging, post-dry-fasting meals, excursions, airport transfers, and follow-up messages at home. I chortled as I contemplated these discrepancies. The entire cost of my treatment, including room and board for two months, was less than what I had paid for one day's treatment at a European clinic. And it had already been far more effective.

Hearing a car coming, I turned. It was Dr. Filonov driving Nora down to swim in the rivulet near the Katun. I had a hunch that he was checking on me every day that I walked, and later on, Nastia confirmed that this was true. "He took on a certain responsibility accepting such a sick American patient, especially when Russian-American relations are poor," she explained. I hadn't considered the gravity of that truth, and it made me feel even more grateful to him for this opportunity. As he passed, we waved to one another, and Nora barked at me.

When I returned from my walk, I took a moment to change into my black yoga shorts, white T-shirt, and worn Birkenstocks. I liked to lie down and rest before the treatments began. It was my turn when I walked over to the clinic room, although there was never any written schedule.

Dr. Filonov patted my head as if I were a child when I lay down on the table for Nastia to massage my arms. I smiled back. We were both strong, independent, nature-loving people who loved dogs. All those commonalities strengthened our bond, even if our ability to speak to each other was limited. I was working hard to follow his protocol, and he was monitoring me attentively. That's all I needed to know at the time; the science itself could wait.

Nastia and I chatted as she worked. I asked, "When do you get to see your daughter?"

"Oh," she replied, "I will go to Barnaul in several days for one night."

"Only for one night! She must miss you terribly."

"Yes, yes, she does, but she is so small, and she loves Dima's parents. It is okay—I have to help Father."

"I understand; I love my father too."

The perpetual chatter in the treatment room made me whimper for solitude, though. The bus driver, Maxim, was camped out on a sofa in the corner watching YouTube videos with the sound blasting on his phone. He would show a juicy clip to patients and make what seemed like crude comments. Patients screamed, unable to bear the massages and muscle injections. *Where can I rest in nature close by?* I wondered as I left the fracas.

Walking no more than a few paces out of the treatment *dacha*, I stood at the top of the stairs that looked over my sleeping porch. There was a wooden ladder going from the porch down to a narrow path that led through tall grasses. The path looked like it meandered a short distance to the bubbling rill and dam that I loved so much. As I stood there, staring, pondering how I could get away from the loud crowd of fasters, I saw that the brook had created an islet.

I had a plan. I raced back to the porch of the *dacha,* pulled my red yoga mat from under my sleeping bag, and grabbed my sleeping bag and my Mayapple Center tote bag. I walked back to the sleeping porch to descend the wooden ladder. I hopped from the low-lying grassy bank to the islet I had spied. It was patched with mud, stones, and pebbles. I set up my yoga mat right in the middle of the dam and river. I accomplished all of this without getting so much as a drop of water on my dry-fasting body. This became my afternoon ritual.

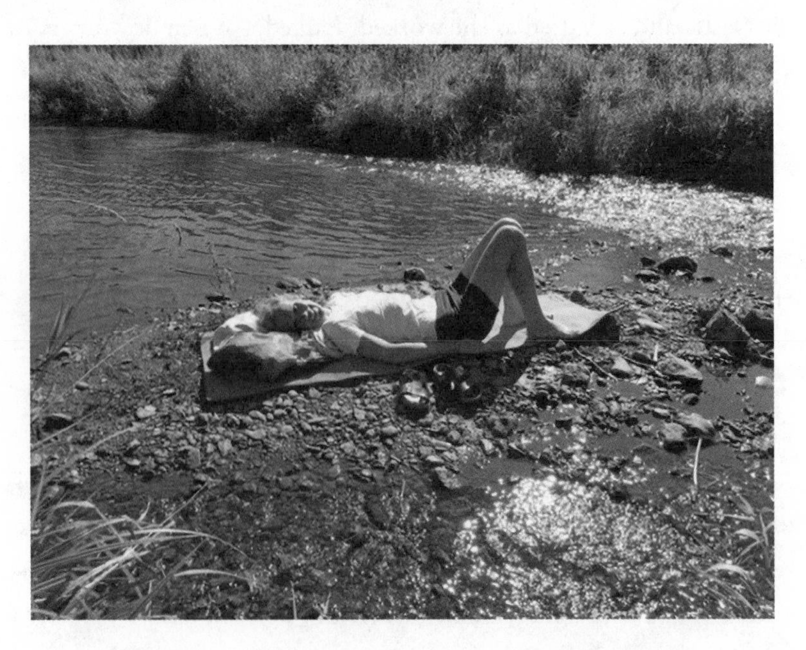

Basking on my red yoga mat on the healing island (photo by Vitali)

The red yoga mat seemed significant. Without it I wouldn't have been able to seek solitude on the damp, pebbly island. I laughed out loud when my mind substituted "yoga mat" for "wheelbarrow" in the William Carlos Williams poem "The Red Wheelbarrow":

> so much depends
> upon
> a red yoga
> mat

My peace depended on the red yoga mat. I lay on it under the sun and rested. I couldn't hear anyone talking, and I couldn't see anyone, although they could see me in the distance if they looked closely from the top of the stairs.

Red dragonflies with burnished sumac bodies and shimmering wings landed near me. The river's rhythmic lullaby softened the tension in my shoulders and chest that stemmed from the treatments, the bus driver's crude jokes, and the bustle of the center. Day one was as serene as could be.

After the sun had set, I ambled to the wooden landing where my sleeping bag was waiting for me; I had dropped it there on my way to the island. I slid my yoga mat back underneath my sleeping bag and camping mattress. My old mountaineering gear was coming in handy in Siberia, for I would have had sore bones without the trusty mattress.

It was time for well-deserved rest, but I hadn't checked in with my critical support group, Siberia! Sweet Siberia!, yet. "All is well. Day 1 was easy. It gets easier the more your body gets accustomed to it. Good night. I am being a wise warrior."

"Wise warrior" was a mantra I devised for myself earlier that spring, dubbed in part for a yoga asana called *Virabhadrasana* in

Sanskrit, or warrior posture. I thought of the inner warrior as deftly navigating life; this is who I wanted to be.

. . .

When I woke on September 12, I was drained from enduring the night noises. The Russians had been loud all night, walking in heavy boots down to my perch and talking around me. I slept restlessly sometime after midnight, but my mind was distracted by the *thromp, thromp* as boots clunked down the stairs, followed by the *Buh deuh da rahhh*, or Russian laughter. I groaned, hoping it would quiet them. Dark thoughts seeped through the carefully constructed filter in my mind that was meant to keep negative energy out. Maybe I should just quit my dry fast and go home where I could sleep? I scolded myself for having thoughts of quitting. I wasn't even hungry or thirsty. *I would be very shocked if I quit on account of not being able to sleep. I want to kill off the diseased cells in my body. Everyone around me is working hard to support me, from Dr. Filonov to my family.* The imprudent thought never returned for the duration of my dry fast.

I found that I slept best in the beginning of the first longer fast, but that sleep was light and interrupted toward the end. I was burning the essential reserves I needed to endure this fast. *What if I can't make it?* When I saw Nastia that morning, she asked how I slept. "*Plokho!* Badly, Nastia. Everyone is so loud." Nastia offered to rent a tent for me when she went back to Barnaul on her day off, and I accepted.

Later in the morning, Dr. Filonov drove me in the rugged Neva to the special meditation site in the woods at the confluence of the three rivers. Dr. Filonov could see straight through my fatigue, and he said that the meditation would energize me. Before we left, Tania was walking by, and she translated for us as he said, "You are a solitary person. You need a quiet place to dry fast. I understand that."

I spent several hours there, visualizing that I was breathing healing white light into my body. When I exhaled, I imagined that I was releasing diseased cells. I would continue this healing meditation every day throughout my fast.

By bedtime, I floated into sleep on a cloud of meditative energy.

• • •

Gray wisps of mist surrounded my chilled cheeks when I exhaled the following morning, so I went back to the *dacha* to put a wool base layer under my yoga pants and pull the hiking pants on top of all of that. D had packed an Irish wool sweater that Dad had sent me in college. That was going underneath the down jacket that had served me well when I was hiking in Patagonia. I was prepared for Siberia with symbolic garments that had seen me through hard times before.

An elderly lady was stretching vigorously outside another *dacha* as I set off for my morning walk. I had heard that she was there with her daughter and that they came every year. After her daily round of Soviet stretches, she and her daughter would walk to the bridge together, and I frequently encountered them on the road. *How impressive they are. If a lady in her seventies can dry fast for nine days, I can surely do it.*

That morning, walking the familiar road felt repetitive, but I made it to my meditation site, where I paused to breathe in the light and do a round of *mette* meditation in which I first repeated:

> May I be filled with loving kindness.
> May I be safe from inner and outer dangers.
> May I be well in body and mind.
> May I be at ease and happy.

Then I shifted it to the second-person pronoun, so I could wish the Russian patients well. They didn't mean to be loud, I figured. They were just struggling to sleep at night while fasting.

Lighter in mind and soul, I trekked on a little more nimbly through the woods, taking a path I had found to reach the bridge. It was a relief to make it around the last bend through the woods and up the slight hill to the center. Some days I wasn't sure I would have the stamina to make it all the way. The gentle uphill gradient brought me to a state of breathlessness when I crested the hill and came up to the big open gate that had stymied D when we first arrived.

While I was resting and waiting for my treatments that morning, I wrote, "Day 3, September 13th. I have no profound thoughts. I hope to survive through day eleven. I have no hunger, no thirst, no pain. I am just tired and weak from not sleeping. I watched the videos on my phone from the first fast. I had so much positive energy that I was brimming. This time I lost it."

Ping.

I stopped writing and pounced on my phone. Back home in the far reaches of Russia, Natasha had texted me, and I copied and pasted it into Google Translate. "Michelle, you cannot have any negative energy on this fast. You have to rest so the body can heal. I know the Russians are loud. Find a quiet place." I knew she was right.

After my treatments, I lay down on my red yoga mat on the island and let the river song wash away my grumpy thoughts. My friend Asif had recommended that I bring Dervla Murphy's *Full Tilt: Ireland to India on a Bicycle*. I hoped to escape into the bicycle ride and feel refreshed, as I had done through reading books all my life. This one sounded promising. It recounted the story of a thirty-one-year-old woman who left Ireland in 1963 and bicycled through Iran, Afghanistan, and over the Himalayas to Pakistan and India. It sounded just like my kind of adventure.

I looked up from the dimly lit page to see that the mountains had become a dark hue of green with stars appearing in the sky above them. I shivered in my fleece jacket and yoga pants. The bulk of the book was now in my left hand, and I was somewhere in Pakistan with Dervla. If she could endure dysentery, heat stroke, filthy food, and flies, I thought I could withstand a few chattering voices in the night in one of the most beautiful and safe environments I had ever been in.

When I was back in my sleeping bag nest, I felt replenished. I fell asleep with visions of Himalayan glaciers and bicycles in my head.

• • •

From the steps of the treatment room, as I waited my turn the following morning, I wrote in my journal: "Day 4, September 14th. How swiftly energy can shift like a seesaw. I slept well, but I was so weak walking in the cold morning air to my meditation site that I thought I would never make it to eleven days. Then, after meditating in Dr. Filonov's special place for me, I was flooded with energy. Whence did it come? I walked back in the sunlight, rejuvenated. Andrei gave me a powerful massage in my painful hips. I CAN DO ELEVEN DAYS!" My hips were hurting either from the walking or from cellular debris shifting inside my body. I didn't know which, and it wasn't time yet to ask for scientific explanations.

At the conclusion of a long day four, homesickness settled into my body like a bleary blankness. I wrote a long message on WhatsApp to Siberia! Sweet Siberia!

> Good morning to you, and good night to me. Today makes three weeks that I have been here. So many days left to go. I am feeling homesick today, as much as I appreciate the

> opportunity to be here with Dr. F. There are some who have made it to day eleven; apart from looking disheveled, one would never know. The way they break the fast is to sit in the icy rill. Lena pours buckets of water over them. The icy soak sounds like heaven after eleven days of no water. You get very hot at the end, they say. The ice water is beneficial for the immune system. Then they drink hot water, and Lena gives them a bright yellow drink that she makes from herbs that help the intestines to start working again. I didn't get to do all of that last time, but I will make sure I get to do it next time. Good night. I love you.

There was no one else to talk to, so I added one last message:

> Though I have survived day four, Dr. Filonov knows I am not as strong this time. He thinks I wasted energy trying so hard on the first fast. I will make the crucial time period. He says I must do it. There is a lot of support here for me.

Janet woke up early that day and wrote, "Thirst and hunger I have not known, but homesickness I know all too well. We will be happy when you are home again." D was quick to build me up. "Just think about the positive things and everything you are doing to heal." I dwelled on that.

Natasha had asked me to send her the same recap message I sent to my family every day so that she could support me too. Now she wrote, "My dear little sister, be strong. It is necessary to find harmony in yourself." I was being fed not with food but with words.

Even so, I had been smiling and joking all through the seven-day fast. This time I must have looked like a contemplative monk.

Just as I was about to attempt another night of sleep, someone came to tell me that Nastia had arrived with the tent from Barnaul. Her husband, Dima, set it up for me a few steps away from my healing island in the river, and I clapped my hands in gratitude, like a pantomime. I dragged down everything I needed to make my nest, along with my journals, phone, and extra layers. I hummed happily as I thought about taking up residence at 1 Tent Lane, Siberia.

I slept in on day five for the first time, relishing the quiet sanctuary of my tent. When I encountered Sergey Ivanovich later, I could tell that he was disappointed that I hadn't walked and meditated before my treatment; perhaps he was worried that I would give up on walking like some other patients had done well into their fasts. I promised I would go in the afternoon. When I lay down for Andrei's masterful liver massage, Vitali told me it would release bilirubin. I hoped that was true, since my bilirubin levels had been inexplicably elevated all summer.

I felt something shift and release as Andrei worked and cajoled my liver over the next hour. I closed my eyes during the cupping phase. *This is my painful healing journey to take. I am seizing the day after spending the last several years in bed. I can endure anything for six more days.* I was groggy afterward, so I lay on my island thinking about how I had turned the corner. Being next to a river while dry fasting is transcendental. I couldn't get enough of the water and its vitality.

I knew I had to start on my walk, although I felt weak from not logging enough hours of sleep over the previous four days. I felt in tune with the sounds and smells of the forest, though. Revitalized by the Katun, I briskly walked all the way home afterward to zip myself up in my tent for the night.

My family was waiting for good news, after the first snarled days of this fast. All the exclamation points I had been using had not fooled them; they could read me too well. "Aloha! I'm snuggled up in the sanctuary of my sturdy Russian tent by the river. I think I am getting all the light and encouragement you are sending me. It was my best day so far." I narrated my fifth day of dry fasting and included a selfie, in which I was smiling in the tent.

My tribe was elated. D wrote back, "Very, very good! You sound so positive! U look great." I fired back, "I'm on my way to a brand-new life!" Janet wrote immediately as well. "Such good news coming from your tent. Keep up your good work and courage!!" From Dad: "The greatest gift for me will be to have you come back healthy!!" Dad thrived on good news. I drifted off into a profound sleep, humming to myself, *On to day six.*

. . .

I woke to the river's melody and sang my fasting song to its beat, lilting upward on the "six" to mark the day I was on. On my phone, I tapped out a tentative question that had come to me during the night: "Would you all consider juice fasting on my day nine in solidarity? I'm going to ask nine friends. Dr. Filonov has said that can be the hardest day, if I understood correctly."

I was gaining energy as the days went by. This was bewildering to me. *I am not eating. I am not drinking, I am walking ten kilometers a day, and yet my energy is now picking up? How can this be?* Much later, I would discover through medical testing that my body had genetic MTHFR defects. Since I had poor methylation, I had a decreased capacity for detoxification. The more I dry fasted, the better I felt. This understanding of the science would come later, though.

On the way back to my tent, I passed several Russian patients sunbathing on the wooden porch. Yoga mats were on Dr. Filonov's packing list, so almost everyone had brought one. Two girls had their heads bowed together and were reciting Russian Orthodox prayers together from a gilded prayer book with iconography. The daughter of the seventy-one-year-old dry faster was sitting in the corner sniffing half an orange, as if it were intoxicating. She must have seen my inquisitive frown, because she held up the orange, so fragrant that I could smell it from several feet away, and called out, "*Aromaterapiya!*"

"Ah, *harasho*!" I called back, dumbfounded that she could sniff the orange without biting into it at this advanced stage in her fast.

Holding court on my island, I turned to my journal, in awe of my physical state. "Day six, September 16th. I have a natural spring of energy. My gait is light, and my spirit is at one with nature. I have walked sixty kilometers thus far on no food and no water. I'm feeling an odd sensation of worthiness today for the first time in eons. I feel eager to finish writing *Soul Mate Dog* and complete revisions on my Kundera book." My mind brimmed with excitement at the surreal prospect of writing again.

I was reveling in the upsurge in my fast. My tribe deserved to know this, so I wrote, "I felt so well on my walk this morning that I walked another five kilometers this evening, for a total of fifteen kilometers." It had been out of the question to walk all summer, and suddenly I was walking without food or water to fuel me? It was uncanny.

"Dad and I and Arthur will fast with you." Their solidarity gave me strength as I prepared to end day six. When I thought about the words "day seven," it occurred to me that I was fasting into uncharted territory, since I had broken the last fast on day seven.

So far, I hadn't contacted anyone but Janet and D, but now I started sending a few tentative messages in hopes of finding a few more friends to fast with me. In a rush of support, fourteen friends agreed to fast with me on different days from Houston to London to

Australia. Among them were D and a few of his colleagues, who were charting my journey. Their solidarity bolstered me.

On day seven, I found strength in the warmth of the Indian summer and solace in my solitude with the lively river as my companion. Janet, an introvert like me, wrote, "When you leave Siberia, I expect you will be jolted by how noisy the world is. Much to be said for being by the water with only sounds of nature. Carry on, little one of enormous strength!"

And carry on I did. At this point, nothing was going to stop me.

When I woke up, my song was joyful. "One, two, three. Four, five, six. Seven, e-i-g-h-t nine, ten, eleven!" I was nearing the mythic ninth day and there had been no crises. I had no pain, no thirst, and nothing was bothering me in my physical body. I had trained for this marathon; I had cleaned enough debris out of my body to sustain this power scrubbing.

D wrote to me as he was preparing for bed in Houston, twelve hours before my time zone: "What you have accomplished so far is just crazy. As in crazy impressive." A well of pride rose in my chest. The word "accomplished" had been banished from my vocabulary for a long time.

Day eight was phenomenal. My fasting friends started sending me photos with their green juices from San Diego, Michigan, and Houston, and it brought me strength. They had all picked random days, which was even better. My childhood friend, Melissa, from Interlochen, sent a photo of a green smoothie with lightning bolt emojis to energize me.

I bounded out on the misty, sunlit morning with more energy than I had had thus far. I walked down a tiny path to a new place by the Katun, an insulated swimming inlet. It was created by a circle of rocks that kept it safe from the current. There, I inhaled the peace of the morning as I meditated. Post-meditation was my favorite time to write to Siberia! Sweet Siberia!

> Day eight. I feel like a gazelle. My energy is picking up as the days go by. I slept from eleven p.m. to eight a.m., for a total of nine hours. I woke up to Dr. Filonov unzipping my tent to check on me. I am supposed to write to him as soon as I wake up, and he didn't like that he hadn't heard from me yet. He finds my ability to sleep on day eight extraordinary; the Russians sleep poorly at the end of the dry fasting. It will be 77 degrees today, but in a few more days, the temperature will drop severely. I can't describe how free and happy I feel.

A master forager, D asked if any of the Russians who had exited from their fasts were hunting mushrooms. "It's a national hobby," he added at the end of his message.

"Yes," I replied. "Everyone is hunting them. Plus, the herbs that grow here are rare and medicinal as tea. Everyone has been picking them, drying them, and packing them. I have no idea what anything is. Must take a Siberian medicinal tea walk with Dr. F." I felt a kinship with the Russians and their fervor for foraging nature's bounty, a skill I'd learned to love in ecology class at Interlochen long ago.

When I walked back to the center and had my treatment, I asked Dr. Filonov why I was feeling so vibrant without any food or water, and he said he had never seen anyone with this kind of energy on day eight. "Father says you must go on the excursion today. It's a very special place," Nastia urged. I had been skipping them because I wanted to conserve my energy. All the other patients had broken their fasts, and I was going on day nine.

We walked down to a makeshift boat launch, and only then did I realize that we were taking high-speed motorized rafts to get there, like the ones typically used for whitewater rafting excursions. The guides outfitted us with lifejackets, and they schooled us about how to rope-in. I was wondering how safe it was for me to be whitewater rafting when I was so advanced in my fast. *Perhaps my reflexes wouldn't be fast enough if we capsized? I wasn't supposed to get wet, but what if water sprayed up on me?* I had avoided even the merest drop of water heretofore. Aside from this, I was game.

On the water, the river's voice was so loud that the guides had to compete with the vociferous current. We were instructed to lean forward and back as the boat shifted from side to side. I didn't understand all the instructions in Russian, so I stayed watchful so I could mimic the others.

The mountains rose up on both sides of the river, and the guides were having fun as they raced north toward the mythical lakes. I didn't understand what was happening when the rafts pulled up to a nondescript section of gravel along the river, and everyone started disembarking. *Where were the lakes?*

Two patients I didn't know very well said to me in rudimentary English, "Are you okay to walk? We have to walk a kilometer to get to the lakes. It's okay. Follow us."

"Yeah, I feel great."

After the guides dropped us off, we walked along a dry riverbed until we came to a clearing where there was an unearthly body of shallow water. I wondered if the words "limpid" or "pellucid" existed in the Russian language. I could see every stick lying under the translucent water. How I longed to immerse my wilted body to plump it up again like a watered plant.

"*Poshli!* Let's go! We are not there yet."

"What? *Sto?* These are not the blue lakes?" I asked incredulously.

"*Nyet. Poshli!*"

As we crested a hill, my breath paused. Just before us was a series of aquamarine pools that were clear to the depths. The blue was otherworldly. Renaissance painters would have envied it and tried to bottle it for their palettes. "Michelle, come!" one of the patients called out to me.

I padded along in wonder.

As I was crawling up a rock to get a better view of the other lakes, I heard squeals and splashing. One of the girls had stripped down to her yellow bikini. She jumped off a rock that jutted over the lake. Others followed behind. Merriment for all. Except for me. Dr. Filonov hadn't had to remind me that no swimming was allowed. He knew I followed each precept of dry fasting.

I disappeared behind a boulder and sat down to lean against a gray rock so that I was well positioned to peer into the mesmerizing waters. I looked longingly at the water, but I maintained my austere discipline. Water would nourish the cells in my body, but we were depriving them so they could continue their sophisticated process of destroying the diseased and compromised cells. There was no turning back from this dry fast. I was all in.

The waters were magical. I felt myself slipping into the etheric realm of meditation easily, and I closed my eyes in contentment.

I heard my name being called in the distance, and knew that it had to be for me, because Michelle was not a name in Russia. It was endearing that the others were so protective of me. Later, I learned that Dr. Filonov had asked them to look after me, but I think they would have watched out for me regardless; I was vulnerable in my state of fasting.

I stood up with my hands splayed out to the sides to see if dizziness would overcome me and, when it didn't, I inched over the rocks until

I was over the crest of the hill where the others were. They were drying off on the sandy shore below, where a few other Russians were cooking a barbecue. Food held no sway over me, but the Russians who had broken their fasts were attracted to the familiar smells of picnic food. *I am in Siberia. I feel good. I am happy. I have had nothing to eat or drink for eight days, and I have not slept indoors once during this time. I am precisely where I need to be. I am healing. I will be well.*

The boat ride back passed in a blur, and when I noticed the tiny gravel inlet by our center, I knew the trip was nearly over. I asked the guide Denis for his number on WhatsApp as we disembarked. I wanted to return to the blue lakes when I could swim, and I was eager to visit the nearby village of Askat, where Buddhists, artists, and yogis lived.

I nearly trotted up the riverbank and across the long field to the familiar dirt road that led back to the center. I glanced back and saw that I was ahead of everyone else by many meters. *I am dry fasting; they are not. I am agile like a wild animal. What is happening? I am not even longing for dear bed, and I have been out on a rigorous excursion.* The sun was setting over the hills as I sauntered down the final stretch of road leading to the center. Dr. Filonov was watching out for my return. Nora came running down the road to greet me, and I patted her head as I heard, "*Horoshaya excursiya?*" I knew he was asking if it was a good excursion.

"*Da, da, ochin horoshoya,*" I replied. "*Bolshoi spasibo. Magiki.*" When I didn't know a Russian word, I tried an English or French one out with a Russian suffix. Sometimes it worked, but whenever I got a head tilt, I knew that it hadn't.

Dr. Filonov was satisfied and smiled. "Our Siberian girl!" he exclaimed. "*Molodetz.*"

Everyone was always saying "*Molodetz*" to me, and I knew it meant "You're tough," "Good job," and "You're brave." I waved and called out my customary good night as I walked down to my tent for the night. "*Spokoinoi nochi!*"

Under the light of my headlamp, I wrote in my journal, "Day eight, evening. I am sloughing off layers of old illness." I stripped down to my T-shirt and underwear and lay on top of my sleeping bag. My body had started to heat up at this advanced stage in my fast. I sent one message to my family, to tell them about the excursion—I knew they'd worried—then, after receiving a speedy, loving message from Janet, I curled up to sleep.

...

When I woke up before dawn on the infamous day nine, I wondered if it would seem harder on this day, but I still felt good. I sent my report to Dr. Filonov. WhatsApp showed me the two tiny blue check marks immediately, indicating that he had read my message even though it was only five in the morning. He must have kept his ringer on to wait for my incoming messages.

Dr. Filonov reminded us frequently that day nine was the most critical day for healing, and that the cells become incinerators on this day that he calls the "acidotic crisis that stimulates cellular destruction." The incineration of diseased cells accelerates and is accompanied by a glow in the patient. The thermometer doesn't record a temperature increase, but the body feels hot to the touch, and the skin is flushed. When I photographed myself in the tent, I could see that my cheeks were rosy, as if I had been posing for an airbrushed portrait. My liver felt hot, and I ran my cold metal external phone battery up and down my chest and the area around my liver to cool down. Since these microscopic cells were intangible to me, though, the epic day nine seemed relatively uneventful.

I didn't realize that it was misting by the time I bundled up and unzipped the tent, so I set off on my walk without much rain gear. It would be one of my last walks on the grand *golodanye*, and I felt slower that morning, as if I were in the rallentando phase of my fast. *Last night may have been the peak of my energy during this fast.*

I divided the road in my head each day. The downward descent toward the field was my first third; I would congratulate myself on making it that far. When I reached the picnic huts and caught sight of the Katun to the right, I was two-thirds of the way to the bridge. The road would begin to flatten out, curve, and meander past the miniscule percolating spring. Finally, I would catch sight of the bridge, where I plunked down to spit out white mucus each morning.

It never failed to astonish me that I was still peeing throughout the day, even on day nine. I squatted in the woods on my return to let out a few droplets of ochre urine. As I walked back, I sang my song over and over that counted off the days I had dry fasted. "One, two, three . . . four, five, six . . . seven, eight, nine, ten, eleven." I added a crescendo and drew out the "niiine," for an extra two triumphant counts. When I saw the wooden gingerbread houses around the bend, I let out a whooshing sigh that I had made it.

Messages started pouring in from my dear fasters supporting me from around the world. My friend Andrew sent a photo of himself in his business suit on the way to work in San Diego, with a green juice in his hand. Some years ago, he had called me in a crisis, wanting to drop out of college. I had encouraged him to march back into the classroom, and later that day, I sent him a photo in which I was holding a teacup with an inspirational message on the tea bag. While I was fasting in Siberia, Andrew paid it forward and sent me an image. He had framed my old photo and I could see my thumb holding up the message on the tea bag. It read: "Happiness is overcoming the most impossible challenge." I exhaled a long sigh of delight when I saw it.

The rain dried up in the afternoon sun. Vitali visited me on my island to tell me that he had spoken with Lena about my exit breakfasts. He explained to her that the porridge was too heavy for me when I stop fasting, and she assured him that I'd only have fruit for breakfast this time. I beamed at him to show my thanks.

Sleep did not come easily, and I was hot. Although I wasn't hungry and would have choked on food if it had been offered to me, given the dryness of my tongue, throat, and esophagus, I started to fantasize about it. I gazed in wonder at a screenshot I had snapped from the *Food & Wine* Instagram account a few months back. The image was the epitome of decadence: a grass-fed hamburger on a brioche bun with melted Roquefort, glazed red onions, and thick slices of white truffles. A vegetarian for most of my life, I would not usually be enticed by such decadent food; this was a D-style meal. Why was I suddenly obsessed with it while dry fasting? *My body is experiencing some primordial sensations. I will just witness them.* I drifted in and out of sleep that night as random thoughts and wants fluttered through my mind.

When I woke up to unzip the tent flap and breathe in the scent of wet pine trees, it was day ten, and I sighed deeply in relief. I felt like I had just passed my dissertation defense. I had breezed through the important day nine. It had been ten days since I had come in contact with food or water. I had made it.

A visceral awareness of the irony of these treatments threaded its way through my thoughts. Dry fasting for too long could have killed me, just as assisted suicide would have, but I had taken that risk, and my heart was beating strongly and steadily.

Valentina had written to me during the night. I knew that she didn't like me sleeping down in the clearing in my tent. She worried that I would be cold. "Valentina, good morning. I am warm and dry in my tent. Don't worry," I texted back. I sent word to Dad, Janet, and Dmitri at once. They were holding vigil and fasting with me. "Good morning, epic lightning and thunderstorm, so I am awake early. Trusty tent is holding up and I am plenty warm."

I confessed to them that I had gotten into trouble the day before. "Dr. Filonov was extremely upset that I made plans to visit the village of Askat with the boat driver. He said that my immune system would be extremely fragile after I broke the dry fast. Everyone got involved trying to translate. It was not good." I felt awful for having offended the doctor. I hadn't understood that I had crossed a boundary by organizing an excursion. I would come to understand his frustration and precautions in the days to come, though.

D wrote at once, "Sending hugs . . . but u do need to relax and let him do his job, as we discussed. It's his job to decide whether to send u on a boat or not." Janet was quick to follow with, "We have forwarded a boatload of hugs. However, Dad says to do as the doctor says for your own wellbeing. Love, D and J."

In closing, I dashed off, "I got the boatload of hugs, and I think they worked. I rested really well, and I am feeling contrite this morning."

I started down the foggy dirt road for my last walk while in starvation mode. Even the smallest pebbles in the road could have sent me toppling. I sat down on a bed of moss to take a respite. While I was sitting there, a German shepherd mix walked through the woods and into my clearing. Observing her from afar, I saw that she was cautious yet hopeful around me. I spoke to her softly in English, reassuring her that it was safe to be with me. I then got up slowly to start walking again, and she followed.

I savored this last walk while dry fasting. I meandered along the misty banks of the Katun and sat by inlets where there were fallen logs or large rocks. The spirited turquoise and white waters entranced me. I could feel that my energy was waning, though. I couldn't have bounded across the field as I had a couple of nights ago.

My new friend sat near me each time I stopped, but not close enough for me to touch her. I wouldn't have petted her, simply because I didn't want to risk getting my hands dirty. I had not, of course, washed my hands for ten days at this point. The dog walked me all the way back to the center. I was so enamored with her presence that I was wondering if I could adopt her and bring her home. *Was I nearing delirium? How would Customs like that at the border? "Oh, I adopted a stray from Siberia, sir."*

I hardly thought that I would cause a ruckus with my new dog, but as I walked down the path to the center, Nastia ran over to shoo her away. "Why did you bring a homeless dog home? They can be very dangerous, you know. You have to be more careful." My new friend was gazing up at me, wondering, hesitating. "I'm very sorry," I said to both the dog and Nastia. "But she was like a morning gift coming out of nowhere." No one was pleased about this gift, so I bade the dog farewell with sad reluctance.

12

A LECTURE FROM DR. FILONOV

As I was turning toward my *dacha* to change into dry clothes, I could see my new friend Kristina walking toward me, the doctor at her side. Their heads leaned in together, as if it were a private conversation. Tall, like Dr. Filonov, she matched his gait. Kristina's long chestnut hair was wound up in a bun on top of her head, and I mused that she could have been a model for the Pre-Raphaelite painters. I hadn't conversed with her while she was dry fasting, but I knew she had come here at the last minute with serious gastrointestinal issues.

Although she was Russian and German, Kristina had lived in London for many years. Her English was the most nuanced of anyone I had met at the center. Dr. Filonov relied on her almost exclusively to translate for me now that she was well into her exit.

Kristina's deep, English-Germanic tone called to me authoritatively. "Michelle, Dr. Filonov wants to speak to you. We will go sit in the *dacha*."

"I just wanted to savor my last walk while dry fasting, that's all." I yearned for a rest after the long walk, but I could tell that something was afoot. *What had I done now? Was it about the dog?*

I sat down on my bed in the *dacha*, where I hadn't slept for a long time. Kristina sat on the bed that faced mine, and Dr. Filonov sat on the bed next to it. The *dacha* was curiously empty, except for us. Dr. Filonov shifted his posture a few times and cleared his voice, signs that I recognized well. He spoke in the voice he reserved for patients. Kristina translated in a tone that mirrored his, in her deep, calm voice.

"Dry fasting is an extremely serious endeavor. I have taken on an immense responsibility with you as my patient because your case is so grave. I want you to go home alive and well. Dry fasting is not a competition, and you need extra time to exit and regenerate the white blood cells. You need extra time for the post-fasting treatments."

What a gift, I thought as I listened. *Kristina is an excellent translator. Dr. Filonov and I would have been at an impasse without her.*

He said that even a nine-day fast had not been a part of his original plan for me. "What I didn't know was how strong your determination was. Your body has a great capacity for this type of healing; this is to be your lifelong treatment method." He smiled as Kristina finished relaying his message.

"Schennikov would let you fast for eleven days because he takes risks that are not medically sound. He is not a doctor." Only later would I learn who Schennikov was. "I was never planning for you to fast for eleven days. I did not want to discourage you by saying no to the eleven-day program. However, you have made a hero's effort." Kristina emphasized the word "hero."

"Letting you believe that you would do eleven days was like a psychological mind game to get you through the critical nine days. He is very pleased, for the healing is profound on the ninth day." She explained that I didn't have the reserves to burn if the liver released another toxic load of residue from the antibiotics; it could damage me. Kristina's voice rose forcefully, albeit kindly, as she spoke these weighty words. As she finished, I heard Sergey Ivanovich mumble something to her, which she chose to translate for me: "He has not slept for the last two nights because he was up *worrying* about you."

I bowed my head, and together, they continued. "You will not be able to have the cold-water therapy in the river. The weather is turning cold now, and this a critical period of rebuilding." I was instructed to start drinking hot water that afternoon and to sleep in the *dacha*. I would be allowed to continue fasting on hot water for two days before I switched to solids. We had discussed that my body wasn't ready for food so abruptly. He preferred tapering with liquids too.

Sergey Ivanovich stood up and paced in the cabin, so I knew that we were coming to a close. I had grown adept at reading his nonverbal cues. "Now you will rest. We will have an exit lecture when you have recovered. I have healed people of serious conditions including cancer, but they didn't always follow my exit instructions when they returned home. You will have to dry fast one day a week at home with great discipline, no matter what the circumstances are. Then, you will also dry fast for seven days every three months. But I will give you all the instructions that you need while Kristina is still here to translate for us. You are very brave, and I am very proud." Having concluded, he came over to hug me.

As if on cue, Valentina came into the *dacha* and handed me my purple thermos filled with hot water. I looked at it in a primal way. I wanted this moment to take place by the stream where I had been sitting for the last ten days, and I walked to it.

Once there, I opened the thermos and raised it to my arid, cracked lips. I cried in relief as I swallowed. I took another sip. Inside my mouth, the water started to dissolve my caked tongue.

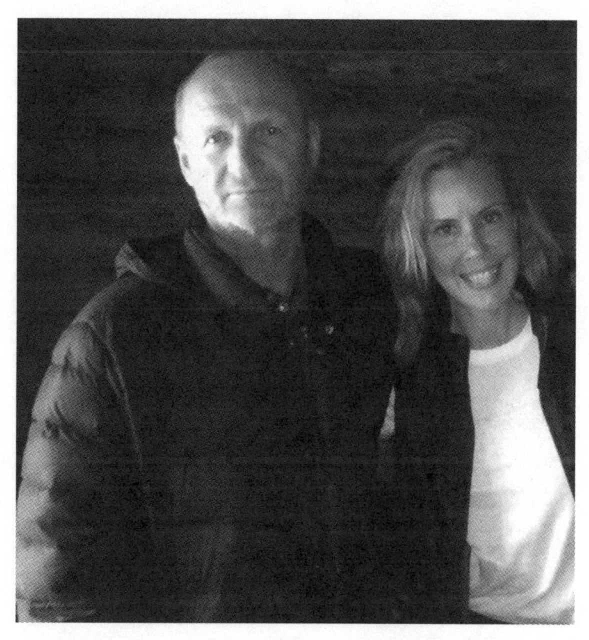

Dr. Filonov and me, after the nine-day dry fast

I sat there on my island, staring at the river as it made its cathartic, soothing sounds.

I was in shock that my fast had come to such an abrupt end. Before I walked up to take a blissful nap in the *dacha*, I took a post-fasting video of myself. Watching it afterward, I couldn't believe how articulate I sounded. I looked like an angel descending from the heavens in some medieval painting, with wisps of sun-lightened blond hair falling out of my bun onto my tanned cheeks. I spoke for several minutes, summarizing Dr. Filonov's lecture and describing how rejuvenated I felt. I did not look or sound sick in the slightest.

I curled up under my sleeping bag for a nap and told my family about the exit lecture. "I have a headache breaking the fast. I haven't peed yet. The body is taking everything. The hot water tastes like life. This is not over. He says the exit is critical and we must get it right."

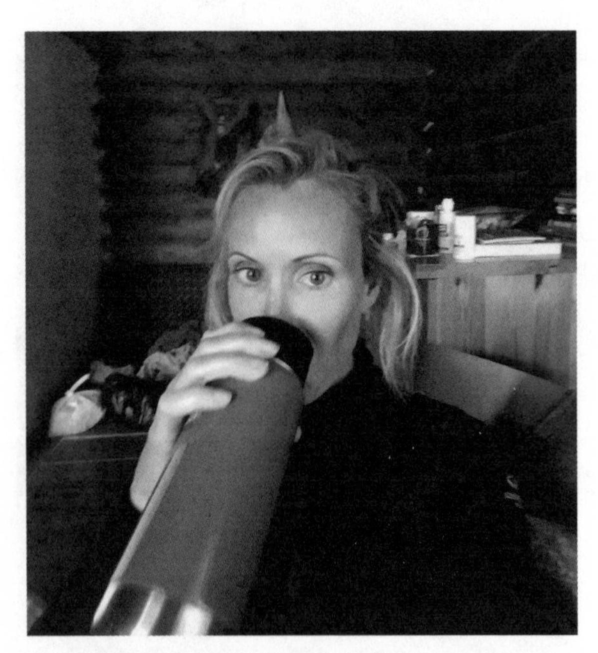

Breaking my Siberian nine-day dry fast in 2017

"I admire what you have accomplished. But Exactly, not over." D had underscored exactly with a capital "E."

From Janet: "Congrats to you for completing this fasting. Each day you will get stronger and continue the rebirthing process. Dad and I are so happy for you. A new person will arrive here in November, healthy, vibrant, and bursting with energy! Carry on, little warrior of enormous strength and endurance!"

To D alone, I wrote, "I feel like I just had major reconstructive surgery and I need to just stay in pajamas and rest." And then, if that didn't explain it, I continued: "The feeling while dry fasting is entirely different than the feeling one has while exiting. I feel serene and strong while dry fasting, but I feel weak and exhausted while recovering." It was a different feeling than the heavy Lyme exhaustion; this weakness felt light and transitory. Although I was still in uncharted territory, hope fluttered around me like the shimmering dragonflies on my islet did.

I knew it was important to mark this day in my journal, so before I surrendered to sleep, I wrote:

> September 21st. It is a day of profound rest. I have much to write, but it must be done later. Dr. Filonov says that the first five days after a dry fast are critical for my immune system, as my body is generating brand-new, strong immune cells, regenerating white blood cells, and creating new stem cells. Although this cellular work is intangible to my naked eye, I can feel that my body is working diligently. My intuition says my body must rest deeply now, including my mind, so I shall put my books and journals away.

13

RECOVERING FROM NATURAL SURGERY

The following morning, I awoke disoriented that I was not in my tent but back in my bed in the *dacha*, with four other girls still sleeping. Rain was ticking like many metronomes on the roof. Other than having a headache, I just felt like sleeping. I had only peed one time since drinking three liters of water. I felt like a camel. Dr. Filonov personally brought me a thermos of hot water from the kitchen, and he cautioned me to refrain from walking that morning.

Lena appeared on the steps of the *dacha* and called out, "*Bania! Gotova!*"

Aha! The bania is ready for me. What a privilege.

The boys had made it steaming hot, and I locked the door. Seated on the wooden bench with my basins of piping hot water, I stripped my dirty layers off, eager to scrub off ten days of dead skin and grime and wash my hair. The water nourished my skin the way the water in my thermos hydrated my dry mouth. The coconut oil had liquified in the heat of the *bania*, and I smoothed it all over my parched body. I even combed it through my hair. I felt human again, not like a wild beast. I wasn't allowed toothpaste yet, so I swirled more hot water around in my mouth and spit it out.

Wiping away the steam, I gazed into the small mirror that hung on the wall by a nail. I gasped at the bones and sinew I saw. I looked like someone coming out of a Siberian camp, and to cover up the image, I stepped into clean blue pajamas. I had been saving them for when I broke the fast. I cinched the dark blue ribbon in the waistband and pulled as I fastened. The bathing ritual sent me straight back to bed.

All was not well during those critical days of rebuilding white blood cells. The water seemed to be carrying things out of my body rapidly. I couldn't believe how I went from feeling energized on day ten of dry fasting, to weak and ill during the seminal period of the exit. I now understood Sergey Ivanovich's furor about my plans for excursions during this critical period of rest. I laughed at my naiveté; the body mandated rest while exiting. I texted the doctor when I woke on the second day of my exit. "I had a brutal headache this morning moving down my face. The pain has returned in the palms of my hands and in the soles of my feet. I feel like I could sleep all day. Did it not work?" I was terrified about that: that after all the fasting, I would find out that it hadn't worked. "Everything will be okay; this is all completely normal. Rest," he wrote back.

Vitali came to tell me how proud he was of me for completing my dry fasts. He would be returning to Italy soon and bade me farewell. "Michelle, the group energy was overwhelming for me, too. I couldn't complete any of the nine-day dry fasts I meant to achieve."

It requires enormous inner strength to dry fast. One knows one's mettle and tests it while persevering through a dry fast.

"Vitali," I told him, "I am indebted to you for all of your support throughout my fasts." I wouldn't ever forget his kindness toward me.

The next day, before bedtime, as my family was waking up, I wrote:

> Good morning, I broke the fast on day twelve with *arbuz.* The watermelon hydrated my mouth. The exit is far harder for me than the dry fast is. I had a "healing crisis" on the night of day eleven with a frightening migraine, dizziness, and ringing ears. This morning, Dr. F said the headache would be gone soon, but that the blood needs time to circulate to the brain after such a long fast.

...

The exit malaise continued over the next couple days. In spite of the treatments I received, I still felt fragile. I reached for my pen.

> I must rest to heal. I feel like a fawn, or like a newly reborn human trying to use its legs for the first time. It has been four days that I have had bits of solid food, and I am still feeling weak with a tension headache. Thus far, I have only consumed watermelon, vegetable soup, salad, and fish soup. Perhaps I just need more time?

That day, Sergey Ivanovich and his team completely overhauled me with medical massage, cupping, circulation therapy, and leeches on my liver. Nastia was about to go home to Barnaul because her fall classes were starting at the university soon. While she was watching the leeches, and I had my eyes closed, we had one of our last conversations during these strange circumstances.

"If you still want to go back to the blue lakes next week, Andrei can arrange it. Did you really like them that much?"

"Oh, I did. I will never forget them."

"You know, the lakes only become blue in September. We come here for the Russian New Year holiday, and it is a tradition for the locals from Askat to swim in the blue lakes then, because they don't freeze over." Her voice was proud.

"Will you miss Altai?" I asked her.

Her blue eyes said she would. "I would be happy to live here all year. But it is not winterized. That's why Father must host programs in other places."

"Ah, I understand. I love Altai too."

I was sent to my *dacha* to rest following the treatments. I sent a message to my supportive team before I drifted off, knowing they were waiting, anxious: "My headache and pains are gone. I am to rest now, and then walk three kilometers slowly tomorrow morning. Your Siberian girl is recovering slowly."

After my nap, Valentina summoned me for lunch, and she triumphantly placed a bowl of broccoli, carrot, and potato soup in front of me. Nastia translated for her, saying, "Dima [a Russian nickname for Dmitri] told me that you love broccoli, so this is just for you."

I hugged Valentina and huddled around my hot soup, savoring each broccoli floret that I pulverized into a juice in my mouth. I thought about how my valiant cells had worked to survive in a Darwinian way, and how they were being rewarded now as I nourished them. I knew these simple meals were an integral part of my healing. *I am grateful.*

Just as I was finishing my soup, Kristina came to tell me that Sergey Ivanovich was leaving soon and wanted to give me my take-home instructions, my personal exit lecture. I returned to the *dacha* with her.

With Kristina's help, Sergey Ivanovich showed me how to do my own liver massage. He even showed me how to do a honey massage, which I had doubts about being able to replicate at home.

"In two months, you are to go into the mountains, where the air is fresh, to repeat the nine-day dry fast on your own." There was a brief conversation between them before she continued, "Sergey Ivanovich understands you have a mountain *dacha* in the U.S. where you can do this safely. Is that true?"

I nodded in acknowledgement, exuding the semblance of nonchalance at the efforts it would take to conduct a third fast at home by myself. But I was reeling inside. This was staggering. *More dry fasting? But the effort has been epic already; is it not enough?* I didn't want to miss her words, so I tuned out my collection of inquisitive thoughts.

"Dr. Filonov said emphatically that the third fast would seal the healing. He said that your mind and your spirit are so strong that you will *fly* after your body catches up."

The doctor's face lit up as he articulated this message, and I could feel myself doing the same—as if we were two fireflies there in the dim *dacha*. No medical professional had ever uttered such an optimistic message to me before: "You will *fly*." This was the antithesis of the American doctors telling me to accept a "new normal" every time my Lyme symptoms worsened.

I marveled at the thought of "flying" being my new normal.

Sergey Ivanovich said I already ate perfectly for my body—80 percent vegetables and fruits and 20 percent high-quality wild-caught fish—so he had no food changes for me. Kristina said he knew I would be vigilant about following the careful diet with therapeutic chewing and modest portions.

While the exit lecture was taking place, Nastia came into the *dacha* to show a text message to her father. It was from a patient in the United States.

Sergey Ivanovich asked her to give me the email address, and he asked me to respond to the patient's questions. "I am eager to help,

Sergey Ivanovich," I said. He sighed and ran his fingers through his hair, looking weary. The long season had begun back in April, with the arrival of the season's first busload of patients, and now the Siberian winter was drawing in.

Kristina explained that patients from all over the world contacted the doctor with questions of all kinds. "They don't respect the time change, and they send him WhatsApp messages in the middle of the night," she explained. I had already surmised that my charitable doctor didn't accept payment for these consultations.

"He is in a very unique position, as the man who can heal untreatable diseases, and he is too altruistic to charge his patients when they ask for consultations. Everyone wants to talk to him," Kristina said.

I knew Dr. Filonov felt an enormous responsibility to help people struggling with illness. At the same time, dry-fasting patients require individual attention, and he was one doctor.

Before he left, the doctor said that in twenty-one days we would see the full effects of this fast. Then, I would be in "phenomenal condition." Twenty-one days. Not so long to wait. Then I'd know if the Lyme was eradicated. Yet, without even having that answer, I could feel a new lightness of being.

"*Ya blagadaru*, Sergey Ivanovich." I botched the saying in Russian but was able to express the sentiment nonetheless.

Smiling, Kristina said, "He already knows that. You exude gratitude from every pore, from every smile."

...

There were only a handful of patients left at the center. As it had turned chilly, Valentina decided we could hold their farewell dinner inside the treatment room. We moved the massage tables to the side, pushed medical supply tables together, and made a fire in the fireplace. I was given a delicious fish soup made with onions, dill, carrots, and potatoes. The others, who had by then been exiting for more than a week, helped wrap freshly caught Siberian fish in aluminum foil, and roasted them with vegetables outside over the fire pit.

During dinner, the Russian patients joined Valentina in singing several traditional folk songs together. I heard an old Soviet solidarity in their voices and thought about how such singing must have strengthened them through those bleak years.

A friendly lady with short-cropped neon-red hair smiled at me as she lent her confident soprano voice. Valentina lifted her head and opened her mouth wide to join in the songs, as if her happiness could finally come out to play after all the hard work of the summer. A guy from Oymyakon, where the coldest temperatures on earth have been registered, radiated joy as he provided the lone baritone voice in the songs, still wearing his navy-blue wool coat and hat and with blushing cheeks as the fire warmed him. "*Oo munia genaaah*." Their smiles grew as they articulated the phrases in unison. The mother and daughter were among the stragglers, and they matched the tone of the collective voice seamlessly. "*Oooh gritsa itsaaahaa!*" This verse was somber, but their intonation was so flawless it sounded as if they had been rehearsing. The table was strewn with cups full of hot compote; the plates were piled high with aluminum foil and fish bones, and I was in the presence of a pop-up Siberian choir. I hummed a few bars of the refrains, which brought cheers, as if I had become their fellow Siberian.

Our good doctor walked in for one last fireside chat, and I listened closely as Kristina whispered his words in English to me. "Tomorrow he leaves, and one can see that he is very, very drained and needs a rest. He said Andrei would be taking you on excursions in the Altai mountains, but he can't stop saying that he is very pleased with the work they have done, together with you." She repeated the last part again, as if to underscore it in case I was incredulous. "Your stem cells will regenerate so that you will be able to write your books. Rest for one month now; the hardest work is over. But he said that it is like natural surgery, and you must not overdo anything. Promise me that, Michelle." I felt close enough to Kristina by this time that I leaned my head on her shoulder in silent thanks.

Before he left, Sergey Ivanovich took me aside and said to Kristina, "I will always be her doctor. I will always be there for her." I had tears in my eyes as I thanked them both profusely, feeling inadequate in my indebtedness. It all felt like a dreamscape.

I walked back to my *dacha*, where Dima and Yuri, another therapist, were keeping the fire stoked. Dr. Filonov had said that night, "No more tent for you. Winter is coming soon, and you need maximum rest now." Kristina told me the Siberian air would chill to nearly 0 degrees Celsius that night (or the low thirties in Fahrenheit) and that snow might frost the trees.

After I burrowed in my sleeping bag on top of my bed, my thoughts turned to my family. I fired off tidbits from the evening as I drifted off: "Everything is so fascinating. Dr. F said if we all train ourselves incrementally to dry fast, then if we start dry fasting when symptoms arise, five days will cure any acute illness."

D couldn't resist exercising his sarcasm. "Just five days? Janet and I were getting prepared to do eleven. U sound very gooda." I realized that dry fasting had become normative behavior for me, but it was still a surreal methodology for most of the world.

• • •

The following morning, Andrei prepared to take all the last patients to the airport in Barnaul. Eager to repay Kristina for her tireless work translating during her own exit, I made her breakfast, including the Turkish coffee she cooed over every morning. We exchanged hugs and emails. After group photos and farewells, the bus left our grounds and Valentina and I rejoiced in our solitude. I was the only patient left. I'd be staying an extra ten days. The other patients had started their nine-day dry fast before I had, and I needed even more time to recover; D and Dr. Filonov had made this arrangement before we left New York.

I could see how exhausted Valentina was from a long season. The washing table was piled high with dirty dishes, and I wanted to help her. I brought a basin of hot water from the *bania* and set to work. When I finished washing the interminable mound of dishes, I set off for a short walk.

A winter person, I relished the crisp autumnal air that whispered promises of snow to come; it was about 38 degrees Fahrenheit and sunny. My daytime attire on top was a wool base layer, down vest, fleece jacket, wool sweater, and big down jacket over all that. On the bottom, I wore every pair of pants I had one on top of another. I never took my fleece-lined purple wool hat off anymore.

They locked the big gate that morning for the first time since D's and my arrival, and Nora began rising at every noise, vigilant and protective like the German shepherd she was.

In the late afternoon, I prepared tea and vegetable soup for us. Valentina couldn't speak any English, and my Russian wasn't much better, but we managed to have fun. We took turns in the *bania* and relaxed by the fire that she built. "I admire how hard you work," I told her. Her brown eyes beamed, and she pointed to her chest and then the sky. "миссия," she repeated. I decided that "*missiya*" must mean "mission," and extrapolated: "It's my mission from God. It's not work." We didn't even need to use Google Translate for that one. The Filonov family astounded me with their selflessness.

The following afternoon, a Hyundai SUV crunched over the stones on the dirt driveway. Valentina pointed and said, "Andrei."

I was surprised to see that Andrei had brought a friend. "Michelle, Sasha," Andrei said, after he had extricated his giant body from the driver's seat and I had given him a hug. "Hello, Sasha," I called out. Sasha had a kind face and a head of chocolate hair; he looked like a much smaller version of Andrei. "I have come with Andrei to translate, but I have, um, not spoken English for a long time. I am rustic."

"Rusty, you're rusty," I said, not to correct him but because I was giddy at the prospect of having a conversational partner. "That's really nice of you. Wow, thank you!" I realized how bubbly and American I sounded.

He gestured to the mountains. "Yes, I am very fond of Altai and thought I would take a short vacation with my childhood friend Andrei to come see you this week. Why not?"

Valentina made a hearty lunch for them that violated every principle of my exit plan.

"Meat! Not for you, Michelle," Andrei quipped.

"All the more for the big Siberian bear." We were back in the rhythm of our banter. After Andrei massaged my legs with the brutal honey treatment followed by a round of cupping, we drove into the mountains toward the markets.

Sasha helped me bargain so I could buy several pairs of tan- and mocha-colored socks patterned with reindeer. It was time to think about stocking stuffers for my indispensable support team. I knew Janet would be charmed by these Siberian yak wool socks. I got freshly harvested honey for Dad. My eyes danced at the Siberian treasures we kept finding. This time, I had stuffed my pockets with rubles, so I splurged on a creamy cable-knit cashmere hat for myself and one for Janet. The sun persisted, but the air turned cold. We were entering the season for cashmere and yak wool. I put my hat on right away and stuffed my dirty purple hat in my bag. Sasha nodded approvingly.

"You look like a Siberian girl."

I laughed and said, "I'm proud to be called that. Thank you."

At the vegetable markets where *babushkas* were selling homemade jars of pickled vegetables, handpicked raspberries, and vegetables from late-summer harvests, I saw a lone grapefruit. "*Russki?*" "*Nyet. Kazakhstan.*" I had been craving grapefruit, one of my favorite fruits, and Andrei and Sasha laughed at me as I forked over a few rubles. "You have never seen a grapefruit before?" Andrei joked.

Back at the center, I squeezed every last drop of grapefruit juice into my cup the same way D did. I had a new appreciation for the way he saved food, "RGO style."

After that day, we fell into a pattern. Andrei would give me treatments, and then he and Sasha would take me out to see some sight. It was kind of them, and I appreciated their efforts to keep me entertained. All the same, I could feel my morale slipping a bit as the days went on. We would eat dinner while bundled outside, and then I'd huddle in my sleeping bag in the cabin at night. I hadn't changed my clothes in a week because I needed all of them. I frequently had thoughts about bathtubs, a toilet, a shower, a mirror, a bed, and clean, fresh clothes. At night, mice would crawl over my sleeping bag, relentless in their nighttime commutes. They had no fear of me at all. I took to sleeping with my wool hat on and my scarf wound around my neck so that they couldn't access my face. My homesickness—for D, for my father and Janet, for familiarity—had become sharp and pointy.

If I had to rely on my memory, I know it would have been fallible when recalling those final days in Siberia, so I turn to my journal again to recount the story:

Today is much better. I had a big surprise: Sergey Ivanovich came back early to check on me. Tomorrow he will work on me himself. I feel a tad stronger today. Andrei gave me a lengthy deep-tissue massage this morning—not a gulag massage at all—for which my body thanked him. I have been begging to visit the village of Askat. After visiting some galleries and a yoga and meditation studio, we walked to a dress shop called Lukomorye, where I met an extraordinary lady named Luba. She is a keeper of Russian culture. She hand-embroiders traditional linen Siberian dresses with ancient protective Russian symbols on them. Sasha told her that I have just come out of a fast, and she said she had fasted once for thirty days on water.

Siberia does not stop surprising me. I am having her make some dresses in vibrant shades of blue and white. Even Sasha was taken with the traditional flax tunics for men and is having a handsome one made in crimson and beige. Luba also rents traditional straw cottages, and they could be the set for a fairytale. If I were to live in Altai, I would settle down right there in Askat, five kilometers from the fabled blue lakes.

The fantasy all ended when we came home, and Andrei put leeches on my liver. Valentina made me a cucumber salad and fish soup to cheer me up afterward. It was sunny, and it brought our chilly clearing to 50 degrees Fahrenheit, or 10 Celsius.

As September waned, I thought, *It's time to leave Altai. I would heal better at home now. It's time to go home.*

October finally came. I could write the unbelievable words in my journal: "I zipped my suitcase and placed it outside for Andrei to take. I have given this every drop of energy I had."

I took a farewell walk at dawn. I heard the words again, whispered to me earlier this month by the full moon, by the birch trees and wildflowers. I heard them in the mist rising up from the Katun's waves. *It is your mission to write about dry fasting and disseminate the method to those who are lying in bed in despair like you were.* I felt a great gratitude as I said my goodbyes to this place—to the Filonovs as well as the mountains and the mighty rivers. I had arrived sick and almost unable to walk. Now here I was, standing by myself, able to smell the scent of the firs on the wind, listen to the birds chatter, and feel one with the world in all its greatness and possibility.

14

LIFE ON THE OUTSIDE: REENTRY

He was mastered by the sheer surging of life, the tidal wave of being, the perfect joy of each separate muscle, joint, and sinew in that it was everything that was not death, that it was aglow and rampant, expressing itself in movement, flying exultantly under the stars.

—Jack London, *The Call of the Wild*

In early October, Andrei and Sasha drove me to Barnaul, where I'd stay at a hotel for two nights before flying home to New York. The drive, on a wintry day, was bumpy and lengthy, although Andrei shortened it with his maniacal speed.

Shed these clothes, buy new ones, take a shower, sleep in a bed. When my hotel came into sight, I bounded out of the car. Andrei and Sasha hugged me goodbye. "Write to me on WhatsApp," Sasha called out.

Dmitri had reserved the honeymoon suite for me in this funky bed and breakfast because the receptionist told him it had the nicest shower, which was his only request. I nearly wept when I saw the heated bathroom floor and the large, round rainfall showerhead in the walk-in bath. It was time for a cathartic power washing.

These clothes had me shuddering. I couldn't take a shower until I went shopping. Armed with Google Maps, I found a shopping mall just outside of the old neighborhood where I was staying. There was an H&M store at the entry. I quickly found two pairs of black leggings, a stylish-looking navy-blue sweater, two white T-shirts, and a cheap pair of black ballet flats. The blaring pop songs accosted my ears and seeped into my unsuspecting body that was used to river songs. The throng of customers conducting commercial activity around me overwhelmed my senses. It felt weird to draw my credit card out of the small Ziploc bag I was using as a wallet. I wanted to say, "Sorry, but I just stepped out of another century," but no one spoke English. After the salesclerk kindly cut the tags off from my new clothes, when I made scissor motions with my fingers, I nearly ran back to the hotel with my bag. I'd been daydreaming about this shower for several weeks.

Ritualistically, I set out my new clothes. I set my toiletries in the shower. I turned on the hot water to let it warm up. Never again could I bear to wear those yoga pants that hung off me now, or the dirty white fleece jacket that I had worn nearly every day in Siberia. I had shed so much already—diseased cells, pain—shedding this sullied clothing seemed the final step. I wished I could have burned it.

I turned away from the mirror when I caught sight of my nude body. My upper body was so thin that I could see protruding bones and the sinew wrapping over my skeleton. I had not died. I no longer harbored plans to commit suicide. My body, though, reminded me of the delicate line between life and death—the brink, in other words—to which dry fasting had brought me. Even though the alluring sound of the hot water streaming down onto the pretty tiles of the shower floor lured me, I turned my eyes back to my body. *Thank goodness Dr. Filonov didn't allow me to dry fast through day eleven. Dmitri will blanch when he sees me.*

I placed a washcloth on the tiles and sat down on it, underneath the powerful showerhead, for long minutes. The hot water penetrated through the layers of permafrost and dirt that I had accumulated in my body. Under the stream of water, I let go of a sort of holding that I had been unconscious of.

My shoulders dropped down from ear level, and a drawn-out "ahhhh" came from my mouth. I hadn't realized how much tension I had been holding by being cold and dirty for these last several days. I scrubbed each body part several times, from my forehead down to each toe. I massaged shampoo into my scalp and tilted my head to let the jets of water rinse my hair before I applied a thick, moisturizing masque and combed it through my hair.

I could not get enough of this shower. I rolled my head around from side to side to let the water beat deeply into my ears and massage my neck. When each one of my finger pads started to pucker and turn pale pinkish white, it was time for the shower to end.

As I dried off and brushed my hair into a French twist, I felt like my healing jumped several levels. Over an hour had elapsed since I stepped into the restorative waters. When I donned the new leggings and sweater, I thought I looked radiant in the mirror. It looked like I was wearing makeup, but I didn't have any makeup. I was naturally shining.

I felt like celebrating. I took a taxi to the center of town, to the best restaurant. The inside walls were stone, and diners were chatting on a very busy Friday night. There were no tables left in the dining room, but they found a place for me at a high bar table for one in the corner of the bar so I could look out and people watch. I perused the menu and found that I could read it in Russian, to my delight. I ordered a Greek salad, followed by grilled salmon and steamed broccoli. I decided to sip a glass of dry red wine too.

A few people from the bar tried to make conversation with me and asked if I was a ballet dancer. I laughed and said I was visiting from the States, which brought some consternation. "What is an American doing in Barnaul?" "It's a long story." I brushed them off and concentrated on my celebratory meal. I even toasted myself, lifting my glass and saying out loud, "*Na Zdorovie* . . . to my health."

It was a night to be remembered. Dry tears of gratitude heaved in my chest as I recited one of my favorite E. E. Cummings poems: "this is the birth / day of life and of love and wings."[1]

When I got back to my room, I eyed my bed. It was a king-sized wonder in which I rolled and rolled, stretching out like a sleeping dog. There were no mice. I could sleep naked—I had to since I couldn't bear to put my dirty pajamas on—and the room was warm without boys coming in and out all night with logs for the fire.

In the morning I woke up feeling like the old carpe diem girl, brainstorming about how I would spend the day. I strolled through a forest of rare Siberian fir trees in the arboretum and explored Soviet monuments in the charming historic district of Barnaul, feeling like I had been unleashed into civilization for the first time. No one was watching me, no one was monitoring me. This was novel after nearly two months of constant, if necessary, surveillance. It felt alien to be in a city again.

My friend Tatiana picked me up at the Moscow Sheremetyevo airport and said, with both affection and her signature bluntness, "You look as feisty as you did at Dartmouth, not like you are dying anymore!"

I twirled for her, feeling like a giddy poster child of health. After our breakfast, my father-in-law, Valentin, came into the café as planned. I had been ill the last several times he had seen me, so his face showed incredulity when I leapt up to give him a Siberian hug. He whisked me home to show me off to my mother-in-law, Nadezda, who also rushed out to hug me before we went for a brisk walk. Nadezda teared up at how lively I was, and I did too.

They are the first ones who get to see the new me, I thought.

When we came in from the cold—one Russian stereotype that has not been broken—I picked up their cat Klara for the first time in years without having an allergic fit. They made me my favorite foods for a celebratory lunch: broccoli and avocado salad with beluga and eggplant. They could not get over my stream of Russian, and I continued the conversation with Valentin all the way to the airport. As I walked from the car to the terminal, I thought, *I am loved. I am well. I am shining and bouncing!*

Deprived of my sense of smell for years, I had forgotten what body odor smelled like. In the airport, though, and on the plane, I wriggled my nose as malodorous wafts offended my nostrils. My post-dry-fasting sense of smell was like a wild animal's. For the first time in years, I experienced no pain on the flight; I was not wincing or shifting my back in the seat.

I bounded toward D at the airport. It did not escape me that I had barely greeted him several years ago on my way home from Istanbul, bewildered at the decaying changes in my body. He grinned and lifted me up in the air. "It worked! Look at you! I can't believe it! It's really true!"

I felt like I had really made it.

I called Dad and Janet immediately. "Am I ever glad to have you back on American soil." Dad sounded like an ebullient puppy. Janet piped up as we chatted. "Hallelujah that our little one is feeling so well now. We are so proud!" This was the best reentry conversation that we all could have imagined.

I could hardly wait to see my best friends in the city. Just two days later, I was meeting Kate for lunch in Gramercy. I arrived at the restaurant first and when she walked in, I raced to hug her. She looked at me with tears in her eyes and said, "I can't believe you did it. It's over. My Miche is back. I'm so happy." These words were the leitmotif to our lunch. Later that day, I met Doug for a walk in Gramercy Park. "You're so attentive," he remarked. "You haven't been able to fully focus on the conversation for so long because of your pain." The rest of the afternoon he kept exclaiming, "We can actually walk around together!" and I kept responding with his old words: "The shipment of hope finally came in."

• • •

Thinking it might be wise to review my progress after dry fasting, I had reserved a spot at the clinic in Europe prior to leaving for Siberia, and it was nonrefundable. The tests that were taken there, three weeks after my exit, were haywire, as Dr. Filonov said they would be, for my blood was still cleansing and my white blood cells were still being renewed. Dr. Filonov had instructed me not to have testing done for six months after a long dry fast because the body is regenerating, and the results would be erratic as cellular debris is leaving the body.

Toxins were still being carried out of my body after this extensive natural surgery, so my basic blood panels were in disarray. My inflammation levels, however, were low for the first time in years. What those tests, and later tests, did show was that the *Borrelia* bacterium was no longer in my body. All Lyme-related tests came out negative. The doctors were dumbfounded.

At the clinic, I overheard one of my doctors saying that all my symptoms would return after this bizarre treatment, and that I was surely still "a very sick girl." One cannot imagine how surprised I was to hear that I was still sick. Did he imagine it was good for my freshly invigorated morale? I had been out climbing mountains instead of lying immobile in a hospital bed, and I had already started to write this book. I wanted to ask him if he had forgotten that all my autoimmune symptoms had cleared in Siberia. My debilitating joint pain had cleared completely and hasn't returned in the four and a half years since. My chronic fatigue, sinus congestion, migraines, and candida: all gone. My chronic back pain was also gone, and it, too, has never returned. Even more importantly, where once I found it nearly impossible to leave 1 Bed Avenue, I now don't even like to lose the time it takes to nap—I'm conscious of having years to make up for.

Years have passed since I overheard the skeptical doctor's remark, and I wish he could see me now, still shining and bouncing. I am hiking and running and playing my saxophone and cello. I have completed a vigorous yoga teacher training program. When I attended a writers' workshop and read from a new manuscript, I didn't lose my words. Nor did I forget what I was talking about, like I used to. I am writing from morning to evening, for my brain is humming again with lucid thoughts.

What's funny is that even while I was at the clinic where I heard the doctor refer to me as a "sick girl," other patients would take me aside to ask what I was doing there when I was so healthy. They all took the shuttle each morning from the hotel to the hospital, whereas I walked the hilly route, morning and evening. The skeptical doctor was correct in thinking that my journey had not concluded, however, for there was more dry fasting to be done.

15

ONE MORE ROUND ON MY OWN

Dr. Filonov had prepared me for the upcoming journey when he told me I would have to repeat the nine-day dry fast at home. He told me that people mistakenly think five or seven days of dry fasting will cure years of illness. "Do not think that one nine-day dry fast can cure years of disease. It could take one to two years for your body to reset completely and rid itself of diseased cells and residues of pharmaceutical drugs. Each dry fast treats an ailment in your body, but all this dry fasting is cumulative. You must have peace, tolerance, and patience." He added, "At some point, you will be healthier than all of your friends."

These words nourished me as I geared up to fast again. Since I didn't want to miss Christmas with my family, I asked permission to start my nine-day dry fast earlier than planned, and the doctor acceded.

In early November, Dmitri drove me to Vermont. Janet flew out of the house to hug me, and then I bounced in to hug Dad.

"TOC! Oh, TOC," Janet sang out, "we are so happy to see you."

"Michelley!" my dad cried joyfully. "I can't get over you. I would never have known you had been sick from looking at you." He beamed with pure joy at the sight of me and folded me into his chest for a long hug. I was home.

"Sergey has proved the world wrong about dry fasting. I am elated to see my beautiful girl come back to life," Dad couldn't stop exclaiming.

We spent the weekend discussing the wonders of dry fasting and Siberia, and I didn't crash on the sofa a single time, which everyone noticed with glee. Janet said, "I have gone from being concerned to being enlightened about Siberia."

D dropped me off in the Berkshires at the end of the weekend. I wanted to be alone and in nature for this dry fast. It passed remarkably well. Even though I didn't have the cupping treatments or massages, I walked outside every day, and I slept in the screened-in porch in my trusty yellow sleeping bag. The more dry fasting I did, the easier it became, and the stronger I felt, although I still experienced moments of discouragement.

A white, foamy mucus lined the sides of my tongue while a thick, lacquer-like pea-green mucus coated the center of my tongue. There were also clumps of yellow mucus lacquered on my front teeth. If an intruder had come to the door, all I would have had to do was bare my tongue and the person would have run away in terror.

On the fabled day nine, which was a Saturday, D joined me, armed with ingredients to make compote. He whisked me up to my favorite spot, Bash Bish Falls, in the Taconic mountains of western Massachusetts for a gentle hike on my ninth day. As our feet crunched on the rust and rouge maple leaves, D put his hand on the small of my back to propel me up the hills. There is something mesmerizing about the energetic effect running water has on those who are dry fasting. We sat on the gargantuan boulders in the shade so I could rest and let the waterfalls put me in a trance.

"I used to romp around the leaves as a carefree child in New England, before the ticks came," I explained to D, for the hundredth time. In this era, I found the miniscule vampires crawling up my legs in search of blood even when I walked on the pavement in the Berkshires.

What irked me was that I had harbored in my body a variation—*Borrelia burgdorferi*—of the same egregious spirochetal bacteria that syphilis patients used to have (*Treponema pallidum*), yet I was out innocuously hiking in the New England woods, not drinking green pools of absinthe cocktails and being promiscuous like some of my favorite nineteenth-century French poets, Baudelaire and Rimbaud. I let those disturbing thoughts go as we walked back to the car.

When we returned home, I checked my phone and found that my entire Russian cheering squad had sent me messages of support, from Natasha and Vitali to Nastia, and even Lena the cook. "I am with you one hundred percent on your day nine," Sergey Ivanovich wrote, bringing me considerable comfort from afar.

"Break the fast at five a.m. with an ice-cold bath, and drink only hot water tomorrow. Pour the large bowl of cold water over your head three times, dunk, and exit the water." Finally, I would be allowed to break a fast with cold water therapy in the safe confines of my own bathtub. It didn't seem nearly as exciting as dunking in the healing Siberian river, but I couldn't imagine D letting me take a dip in the Housatonic river in November.

We set the alarm for 4:50 a.m., and I closed my eyes. Anticipation hummed in my chest so loudly I didn't know if I would be able to sleep over the buzz. I hadn't known if I'd be able to sustain such a long fast on my own, but it had been far easier on the second round.

I jumped up at the sound of the alarm and drew an ice-cold bath. D boiled spring water for me. He came back up with a thermos and mug of hot water just as I plunged into the freezing water. As I poured the water over my head, I couldn't get enough of it. D brought my squeals of delight to an end, saying, "I think that's enough. Let's not overdo it." I clambered out compliantly and wrapped a towel around myself as D handed me the aquamarine ceramic mug of steaming hot water that reminded me of the Katun.

I had tears in my eyes as I stood and sipped the life-sustaining water. My great reward for this hard work. I went back to bed for an early morning nap. *I did it. I can do this. This is my way of healing.* D sent a message and photo to Dr. Filonov on my behalf, and we received a "Bravo" back immediately.

The exit was entirely different than the ones I had experienced in Siberia. We drove home that evening and by the next morning I was up and about with imperceptible discomfort other than the tinnitus in my ears. I knew that this was just a temporary exit tinnitus; it would fade out as I rehydrated. As I drank, the mucus on my tongue slowly ebbed over days to reveal a shiny pink tongue. When I showed it to my old naturopath Dr. Anthony Salzarulo in New York City a few weeks later—whom I visited only to share my successes—he said with great pleasure, "You got a major upgrade in your internal terrain!"

A relaxed fatigue wafted over me for several days, like the recovery period after a marathon when one has made valiant efforts. I asked Dr. Filonov about this improvement in my exit, and he explained that the exit would be significantly less painful with each successive dry fast.

. . .

I had arrived in the land of the healthy people, and it felt good. What would I do with this gift that made me forget my mortality? I started to write again mere days into the exit, for the dense fog had burned off from my brain. The headlights of my neurons enabled me to see my own ideas again.

I thought of the journal entry I had written in Jackson Hole two years ago: "What can be written on a blank slate when one doesn't have the crit-theory brain, the music brain, the lit brain that one once had?" I hadn't known it was possible to get one's brain back, but my music brain, my crit-theory brain, my writer's brain was back. I was no longer in the body of the other. I had a lot to write on the blank slate.

PART III

THE SCIENCE OF FASTING

16

THE FOUNTAIN OF YOUTH IS WITHIN

Everyone has a physician inside him or her; we just have to help it in its work. The natural healing force within each one of us is the greatest force in getting well. Our food should be our medicine. Our medicine should be our food. But to eat when you are sick is to feed your sickness.

—**Hippocrates,** *Hippocratic Corpus*

My complex case of late-stage Lyme illustrates a remarkable irony: the pharmaceutically driven medical industry encouraged me to put high doses of harsh medications and supplements into my body over a long period of time to no avail, while what ultimately saved me was putting absolutely nothing in my body.

The principle at work here was elegantly stated by Nobel Prize–winning biologist Yoshinori Ohsumi in his banquet speech: "Life is maintained by a delicate balance between continuous synthesis and degradation. I found that degradation is just as important as synthesis for the maintenance of dynamic biological systems like the body." However, physicians and nutritionists fail to heed the ancient Hippocratic wisdom that "to eat when one is sick is to feed the illness." Although every doctor is familiar with the Hippocratic oath to uphold ethical standards while practicing medicine, few doctors heed Hippocrates's invaluable medical wisdom about the internal physician each of us has in our body.

Yet we need to awaken that physician within more than ever. Although only 35,000 cases of Lyme disease are reported to the CDC annually, an estimated 476,000 new cases of Lyme and tick-borne diseases are diagnosed annually in the United States alone.[1] A Johns Hopkins Bloomberg School of Public Health report states that Lyme disease costs the U.S. health care system a staggering $712 million to $1.3 billion per year.[2] Patients are not getting well, and there are more of them every year.

As many as 63 percent of Lyme patients experience chronic Lyme, a condition many doctors do not recognize. The lead researcher of the Johns Hopkins study, Dr. John Aucott, said, "These patients are lost. No one really knows what to do with them. . . . There's not a magic pill. These patients already got the magic pill [antibiotics] and it didn't work."[3] How can one get used to a new normal of chronic Lyme in a broken-down body? I'm hardly the first Lyme patient to consider assisted suicide. A study published in the journal *Neuropsychiatric Disease and Treatment* estimates that 1,200 suicides per year in the United States may be attributed to Lyme disease, as a result of depression-inducing inflammatory cytokines, coupled with despair.[4]

Autophagy and Its Role in the Fountain of Youth

Were it not for the synchronicity in my discovery of Dr. Filonov's work while I was lying in bed planning my trip to my final destination, the Swiss assisted-suicide clinic Dignitas, I would never have found this elusive fountain of youth. Hippocrates and his colleagues explained it in the *Corpus* that they wrote and passed down to us from the fourth century B.C.E. This force is called autophagy, a term coined in the mid-nineteenth century by French physiologist Anselmier, which means to consume one's own diseased tissues and cells. Dr. Filonov writes and speaks of the autophagy that takes place while dry fasting; it is his life's work.

I hope that the science of dry fasting can save fellow Lyme patients from the fate that was almost mine. Though my Ph.D. from Johns Hopkins is not in the realm of the sciences, I have conducted extensive research on this subject. I aim to elucidate the science of dry fasting and dispel myths and misconceptions, using myself and others as clinical evidence.

When I wanted to understand the intangible process of autophagy taking place deep inside my body, I asked Dr. Filonov, "What do I read?"

"Start with Ohsumi," he said. Japanese scientist Yoshinori Ohsumi won the Nobel Prize in Medicine in 2016 for his discoveries on autophagy's role in the human body to degrade and recycle cells, which has opened the floodgates for research on fasting and artificial stimulants to cure diseases.

Dr. Ohsumi's work builds on Nobel Prize–winning scientist Christian de Duve's discovery of the lysosome, the organelle responsible for degrading damaged cells. De Duve discovered the cellular container, or vesicule, that transports cellular waste to be destroyed.

He named it the autophagosome. Ohsumi then discovered the process of autophagy in yeast cells, proteins, carbohydrates, and lipids. Ohsumi's experiments proved that if yeast cells are starved, autophagy accelerates to recycle cellular material, so that the organelles, or compartments within the macro structure of the lysosome, prepare cellular waste for degradation. This breakthrough in his research led Ohsumi to isolate the genes related to autophagy. Ultimately, Ohsumi linked disruptions in the cellular functioning of autophagy to aging-related diseases such as Alzheimer's, diabetes, Parkinson's, and cancer.

The American response to Ohsumi's research has largely centered on creating pharmaceutical drugs to trigger autophagy and cure diseases. Dr. David Perlmutter, dean of the School of Medicine at Washington University in St. Louis, responded to news of Dr. Ohsumi's Nobel Prize in the *New York Times* by saying that premature aging, cardiovascular disease, and cognitive decline are the result of having a compromised system of autophagy. He lauded Dr. Ohsumi's work that would lead scientists to develop drugs to stimulate the system of autophagy, yet he mused that Dr. Ohsumi's work has implications that are "the stuff of science fiction."[5]

As I write this, new companies are being launched and backed with millions of dollars to create pills that would harness the power of autophagy and destroy harmful pathogens, excess protein deposits, and organelles. Their endgame is to reverse diseases associated with aging, most notably Alzheimer's. By attempting to recreate the natural process of autophagy in the body, they've missed the brilliant Hippocratic (and Filonovic) point: the body is the healer, and it requires no outside help. The body has the innate capacity programmed into its DNA to heal of its own accord, without outside stimulus of any sort, but the simplicity of this solution has eluded these seekers.

Fasting for Therapy: A History

We have long sought to preserve our youth in Western culture. Remember Ponce de Leon's quest for a mythical fountain? How about Oscar Wilde's novel about the sordid picture of Dorian Gray that aged, while the character's flesh remained uncannily well preserved? Today, we inject Botox in our faces to ward off wrinkles; we inject stem cells in the hopes of rejuvenating our bodies. Yet the body has known how to rejuvenate itself since the beginning of time.

Fasting is referenced in Ancient Greek, Tibetan, Indian, and Middle Eastern early writings as a potent technique to prevent diseases, strengthen self-discipline, and heighten spiritual practices. Moses, Ezra, Jesus, and Apostle Paul dry fasted. Plato, Aristotle, and Pythagoras fasted, presumably on water. Hippocrates, the father of medicine, prescribed fasting, as did subsequent doctors Galen and Paracelsus. This ancient practice can treat many diseases today.

Early fasters in the United States nearly stumbled on it before the fledging American Medical Association (AMA) and budding pharmaceutical companies stamped out research on fasting by labeling it as unorthodox and dangerous. Recently, though, the early wisdom of fasting in America has been returning to the mainstream, thanks to scientists' research at Johns Hopkins University and the University of Southern California.

There's been talk on the street about intermittent fasting since anti-aging expert Mark Mattson, head of the neuroscience lab at the National Institute of Aging and a Johns Hopkins professor, gave a popular TED Talk in 2014 on caloric restriction to promote longevity. The talk, titled "Why Fasting Bolsters Brain Power," has garnered more than four million views.[6] Elsewhere, Dr. Mattson describes his own long-term practice of intermittent fasting. To reap the benefits, he advises eating within a restricted eight-hour window every day.[7] The practice has since gained wide traction.

Dr. Mattson argues that caloric restriction slows down the aging process of the immune system. I propose that intermittent fasting will not suffice; otherwise, there would be far more successful case histories. Extended fasting for medical purposes has met with historical resistance in the United States, though.

Fasting research was thwarted by the newly emerging AMA, in alliance with the emerging pharmaceutical industry in the early twentieth century. French documentary filmmaker Thierry de Lestrade unearthed a fascinating long-forgotten history of therapeutic fasting in the United States, which details how the practice was thriving in the nineteenth century. As he writes in *Le jeûne, une nouvelle thérapie?* (Fasting, a new therapy?), de Lestrade discovered that the disappearance of fasting centers had nothing to do with the treatment's therapeutic effectiveness; it was the consequence of a war led by the medical establishment and the pharmaceutical industry. Fasting was stamped out by the end of World War I, led by the head of the nascent AMA, Nathan Davis, who said that doctors who advised fasting were sapping the base patients of pharmaceutically based doctors.[8]

Yet therapeutic fasting had great success in the nineteenth century, even among doctors. In 1877, Dr. Edward Dewey was faced with the crisis of treating his three-year-old son's life-threatening case of diphtheria. Dr. Dewey made a bold decision to put him on a water fast, a treatment he had seen cure another patient of a severe gastrointestinal disease. The child recovered completely. Dr. Dewey, having become a major proponent of fasting, started a fasting school that attracted many followers, including Bernarr MacFadden.

MacFadden founded a successful Healthatorium in Battlecreek, Michigan, though he was a self-made fitness guru, not a doctor. One of his most famous fasting patients was the writer Upton

Sinclair, who wrote a popular book, *The Fasting Cure*. The book became famous worldwide, influencing early researchers and practitioners of fasting in Russia.

If it weren't for Sinclair's book, Dr. Filonov may not have discovered dry fasting. Here is the path the book took to reach him: A Russian intellectual and close friend of Leo Tolstoy named Sergey Nikolaev received an English copy of Sinclair's book. He put both of his boys on a water fast when they were toddlers. One of them, Yuri, grew up to become a famous doctor at the Moscow Psychiatric Institute. Never having forgotten the treatment that saved him from early childhood illness, the doctor became an advocate of the practice. Eventually, and despite much governmental skepticism, he succeeded in supervising more than seven thousand patients as they conducted thirty-day water fasts. Through his case histories and his books—which have not been translated into English—including *Голодание ради здоровья* (Health through fasting), Dr. Nikolaev influenced current dry-fasting proponents, including Dr. Filonov. His successes were nearly supernatural. When one catatonic patient started talking on day six of a water fast and was ultimately cured of mental illness, Dr. Nikolaev said, "It was the most beautiful day of my life."[9]

When asked what the most important discovery was of the twentieth century—television, radio, or atomic energy—Dr. Nikolaev responded, "None of these. In my opinion, it's the capacity to regenerate oneself physically, mentally, and spiritually by fasting."[10]

Sinclair wrote his book partially so that scientists could conduct further research on the medical benefits of fasting, like Nikolaev ultimately did. As the pharmaceutical companies profited from the sales of medications that they pushed onto patients through doctors, no one in the medical industry was interested in conducting research on fasting, which would never be lucrative for anyone. Had research about fasting caught on in the United States, as it has in Russia, we might not be in a position of spending more than $1 billion a year treating diseases like Lyme.

Instead, the AMA launched a new branch in 1906, literally called Propaganda Department, to root out non-allopathic health practitioners. The director, Morris Fishbein, never graduated from medical school; nor did he practice medicine, but he went on a decades-long witch hunt to discredit naturopaths, chiropractors, homeopaths, and fasting experts. On his list of targets was Upton Sinclair, Bernarr MacFadden, and the famous naturopath Herbert Shelton.[11]

Despite being subjected to FBI investigations for practicing fasting against the directive of the AMA, Shelton treated patients with serious diseases for decades at his fasting clinic in San Antonio and demonstrated tremendous success in his results. He conducted over 35,000 therapeutic fasts during his lifetime. Out of this number, three patients died, all from circumstances that were beyond the doctor's control. One patient insisted on continuing a fast in spite of Dr. Shelton's assistant's insistence that he break it; two others did not follow his protocol. How many medical doctors can say that they lost only three patients out of 35,000, and that the remainder experienced remarkable recoveries?

Shelton was on the verge of discovering dry fasting, for he writes in his book that he watched some patients fast for two to three days without consuming water, because they had no thirst. If he had continued experimenting with lengthening the time of the waterless fasts, he surely would have realized the latent power of autophagy.

Nonetheless, Shelton understood why other doctors shunned fasting: "Few doctors of any school know enough about fasting to conduct a fast with confidence. They prefer the eliminating diet in all cases because their ignorance is so great of the superior method. A few of these men succeed in camouflaging their ignorance and inexperience behind the pretense that fasting is dangerous."[12] We could have surpassed the place we are today in the United States and avoided the crises of overburdened livers that have been exposed to hundreds of pharmaceutical drugs, if we had followed the clues left for us from these early pioneers.

A Time and Place for Pharmaceuticals

This is not to cast doubt on the efficacy of pharmaceutical drugs. Pharmaceutical inventions in antibiotics and vaccines have produced significant health results that have been said to reduce infant mortality rates by 50 percent and reduce maternal deaths related to childbirth complications by 90 percent.[13]

Still, any good thing can be overdone. And as early as the 1950s, critics were warning the American public about the dangers of marketing and overusing medications. The writer John Lear took on this topic in an article called "Taking the Miracle out of Miracle Drugs," published in the *Saturday Review* in 1959. In it, he noted that "prescription of antibiotics without a specific cause for such treatment has reached disturbing proportions."[14] Lear warned that doctors treated symptoms with antibiotics without investigating the origins of the diseases, thereby masking serious diseases with medications.

Lear made the prophetic statement that the overuse of antibiotics would lead to the development of dangerous strains of antibiotic-resistant bacteria. He exposed an advertisement by Pfizer for a new antibiotic that claimed that numerous doctors had found the drug "highly effective" and "clinically proved."[15] The ad was accompanied by the reproduction of doctors' business cards. Lear had telephone operators try the numbers and found that they were all false numbers.

• • •

Pharmaceutical drugs create debilitating side effects. What processes the pills? The faithful liver. Chronic Lyme patients carry a high toxic burden; thus, paradoxically, the medications render many patients even more ill. The liver is already processing pollution, pesticides, chemicals in our food, unhealthy foods, alcohol and caffeine, heavy metals, and mold, among other unidentified substances. The added toxic burden from antibiotics is what contributes to the breakdown in autophagy.

The vast vitamin industry also contributes to liver toxicity by marketing vitamins and supplements that are hardly regulated; chronically ill patients tend to self-medicate with supplements in the hopes of getting better if they can just find the right vitamin cocktail. Instead, their livers become even more overburdened and the elegant process of cellular degradation screeches to a halt.

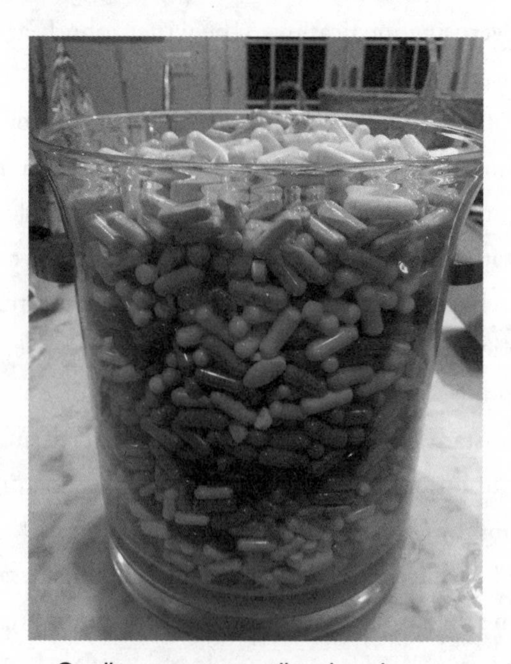

Goodbye, prescription pills and supplements

Dr. Filonov writes that whereas penicillin was a miracle medicine when it was first introduced, the current generation of diseases is more resistant to antibiotics, just as Lear warned.[16] Although Dr. Filonov does not oppose prescribing drugs, he recommends them only in acute cases. In less severe instances, the patient should mobilize his internal reserves in the process of autophagy.

Dr. Ohsumi and Dr. Filonov have never met, but they've been doing similar work for decades: one with yeast cells and one with human patients. Dr. Filonov says that while patients are dry fasting, diseased cells incinerate themselves in a natural elimination process.[17] Dr. Ohsumi shows that the cell encloses itself in a membrane and self-destructs through a recycling compartment, or lysosome, because cells are naturally programmed to die at some point and replace themselves through apoptosis. This is the body's natural cleansing process, but when this system breaks down—because of an overburdened liver, which is Dr. Filonov's explanation for my case, or a high toxic load—then diseases become chronic and nearly ineradicable.

Dr. Ohsumi started his work with yeast cells and then demonstrated that similar processes exist in human cells, although this next stage has yet to undergo clinical trials. Meanwhile, all along, Dr. Filonov has been guiding patients through this process of autolysis stimulated by extended dry fasts, which have resulted in innumerable healings from multiple diseases.

Remarkable Successes in Fasting despite Opposition

The *Los Angeles Times* documented Dr. Yuri Nikolaev's water-fasting successes in an article published in 1972 called "Soviet Cure-All: Eat Nothing for 30 Days." But that didn't lead to a rise in water fasting in the United States, where it is still considered dangerous. Dr.

Nikolaev's work certainly caught the eye of a young medical student in Siberia named Sergey Ivanovich Filonov, though, who comes from a long line of medical doctors.

Dr. Filonov experimented on himself to perfect the methodology and found that his memory and concentration improved when he fasted on water. After he graduated from medical school, he became the medical director for twelve years at the famous clinic Goryachinsk on the shores of Lake Baikal, which was featured in de Lestrade's 2012 film *The Science of Fasting.*

At Goryachinsk, patients practice extended water fasting under medical supervision to cure illnesses, but Dr. Filonov found over the years that symptoms abated after water fasting, only to return later. He attributed this to the increasingly chemical nature of the world.

Dr. Filonov's first forays into dry fasting came from watching his dog dry fast for seven days in a dark shed after she was hit by a motorcycle. On the eighth day, she began to eat and drink and returned to full health. Dr. Filonov researched animal behavior and devoted a large section of his first book, *Dry Medical Fasting: Myths and Reality* (which has not been officially published in English), to show how various animals in the wild refrain from eating and drinking when they are injured or sick as a curative practice.

When Dr. Filonov fell through the ice in an ice-fishing accident just afterward, he emulated his dog and dry fasted. After five days, he made a full recovery. This episode was the beginning of the studies on dry fasting that would lead him to the expertise he has today. He studied all those who preceded him, beginning with the odd case of Johannes Schroth.

Schroth accidentally discovered modern dry fasting in Austria in the nineteenth century by refusing to feed his horses that had fallen ill. After three days, they recovered, so he tried it himself with great success. He became a well-known naturopath who treated his patients with dry fasting.

Another important figure here is Porphyry Ivanov. A mystic, he experimented on himself in nineteenth-century Ukraine to tolerate extreme temperatures, starvation, and ice-water immersion—along the lines of the modern-day phenomenon Wim Hof—until he underwent two weeks of dry fasting. Ivanov had hundreds of followers when he died in the 1980s. Ivanov espoused that fasts must be conducted in natural environments, outside of polluted cities. He recommended special breathing techniques to increase oxygenation in the body, cold-water baths, and long walks in nature. He argued that negative thoughts contributed to diseases. What Ivanov intuited and practiced is not far from the modern practice of dry fasting, even though he was an uneducated layman. He dry fasted regularly on Mondays, Wednesdays, and Saturdays, encouraging his followers to do the same. Ivanov paved the way for Russian medical research in the area of dry fasting.

Although autophagy is studied in the most sophisticated laboratories, from Japan to the United States, those who have practiced dry fasting the most have had little to no medical training, with the exception of Dr. Filonov. Leonid Schennikov, the folk healer from whom Dr. Filonov learned to dry fast, conducted dry fasts at his center in Kislovodsk for more than fifty years until his death in 2019. The only holder of a Russian patent in dry fasting, Schennikov called dry fasting the "method of bodily recovery," according to Dr. Filonov. Schennikov maintained that if one faithfully practices dry fasting, no disease is incurable.

Dr. Filonov would disagree, as he has seen advanced cases of cancer resist the power of dry fasting. Dr. Filonov begs his patients to come to him when they *first* experience symptoms of disease, rather than as a last resort after having exhausted all conventional and allopathic resources. Dr. Filonov doesn't make categorical claims about what dry fasting can accomplish, because each body reacts differently based on its unique circumstances; he doesn't want anyone to think dry fasting is a panacea.

Before Dr. Filonov started treating patients with dry fasting, he underwent a nine-day dry fast at Schennikov's clinic, followed by a ten-day dry fast on Lake Teletskoe in Siberia. He developed his own technique, assimilating local folk medicine with his vast medical knowledge. He then opened his own clinic in the Altai mountains. Through his patient research, experimentation, and practice with thousands of patients, Dr. Filonov has become the world's foremost expert and clinician of dry fasting.

17

THE CHALLENGE OF AUTOPHAGY IN A CHEMICAL WORLD

The process of autophagy breaks down when the body is faced with an overwhelming onslaught of chemicals. The liver cannot cleanse effectively in the modern world on its own, Dr. Filonov argues. We are exposed to thousands of chemicals that our ancestors did not encounter. "Our bodies are oversaturated with poisons of modern civilization. The body's energy is spent on removing these toxins," Dr. Filonov says.

In cities, the body absorbs toxins from pollution and from inhaling gas fumes. Hair dyes and hair spray are toxic, along with house paint and everyday cleaning products. The pesticides and hormones found in foods today are poisonous in the human body. Modern diets with processed foods have contributed to this grave epidemic. Excess toxins from the environment and foods we eat reside in the body's fat tissues.

As the poisons accumulate, they affect vital organs and leave us susceptible to contracting viruses and diseases. As a chronic Lyme patient with high heavy-metal levels and mold toxicity, I constantly felt like I was full of sludge, even though I was adhering to a clean, organic diet. Dr. Filonov advocates for everyone to dry fast, for the body cannot cope with what he calls the "avalanche of modern toxins."

A Growing Epidemic

In *Toxic*, Dr. Neil Nathan, a Lyme specialist, writes how his training to be a family physician did not prepare him for complex medical problems today. "As our world becomes increasingly toxic due to the prevalence of chemicals, heavy metals, genetically modified foods, radioactivity, and electromagnetic radiation, we are beginning to realize that this is a growing epidemic."[1] A few continents away, Dr. Filonov says the same thing. I call these conditions "the mystery diseases," and they include chronic fatigue, Lyme, and certain autoimmune disorders that simply don't respond to treatment.

I posit that the mystery behind chronic Lyme is simple and solvable. Individuals with a genetic profile like mine—which has methylation deficiencies that inhibit the body from naturally detoxing—are at a disadvantage when combatting spirochetes. There is no way to avoid fasting, because depriving the body of its external nutrient or power supply is the key to igniting the process of autophagy. Dry fasting eradicates accumulated waste across the entire body, and as a result, chronic fatigue, inflammation, and brain fog will vanish. It's that simple. "Dry fasting is natural surgery," as Dr. Filonov puts it. It's like chemotherapy without the harsh side effects.

Yet with all the fear surrounding surviving without water, who dares to try it? Many friends have said to me, "Michelle, I would try water fasting, but I think the dry fasting you do is a bit extreme." To this, Dr. Filonov would respond, "Dry fasting is far more effective than water fasting." I believe I have proven with my own body that dry fasting isn't dangerous when you observe the protocols.

Combatting Inflammation from the Inside

What is happening in my body when I dry fast? My body burns glucose and protein rapidly, and then it starts eating fat and abnormal cells; meanwhile, vital organs are preserved and nourished by the accumulated reserves. The body is not only able to build tissue—it's also capable of destroying it. The body immediately leaches toxins from the reserves in the adipose fat tissue.

With water fasting, the body uses the exogenous water, or the external water that one drinks, to cleanse the body. In contrast, when dry fasting, the body uses the endogenous water—or internal water inside the body. That is how we arrive at Dr. Filonov's image that seems like science fiction: "During dry fasting, each cell, in the absence of an external water supply, turns into a mini-furnace—or thermonuclear device—so that only the strongest, healthiest cells survive. The heavy, dead water in the body is cleansed during the dry fast." What Dr. Filonov is calling "heavy, dead water in the body" is inflammation.

In *Toxic*, Dr. Nathan explains:

> The underlying theme for all of these conditions, whether they are triggered by toxins or infectious agents, is inflammation. Toxins and microbes stimulate the immune system to produce inflammatory cytokines, which are messengers used by the body to regulate the immune response. For reasons we are slowly beginning to understand, the body

> is unable to turn off this inflammatory process once it is stimulated by these specific causal elements. What begins as a normal, healthy immune response over time develops into an out-of-control chronic illness. Think of it as a warming campfire on a cold night that erupts into a devastating wildfire.[2]

The way to fight the wildfire in the body is through dry fasting. Dr. Filonov states that inflammation cannot exist without water. Any area of the body that is inflamed is swollen with water. Watery environments are the only places where microorganisms, microbes, and viruses can spread in the body. Hence, depriving the body of water is fatal to inflammation. It's only in a dehydrated state that pathogens and inflammation can be eradicated. The healthy, strong cells survive in the dehydrated environment within the body, whereas viruses and bacteria do not.

Dry fasting releases glucocorticoids, the hormones responsible for metabolizing carbohydrates, proteins, and fats, which provide tremendous anti-inflammatory effects throughout the body. As we age, and as we become overburdened with toxins from the environment or substances we put in our bodies, our bodies struggle to kill off bacteria and viruses. We end up in a low-grade systemic state of inflammation, which dysregulates our immune systems.

Regeneration of Cells—Rebuilding Immunity

Dr. Filonov has found that white blood cells and stem cells regenerate during the rehydration period after dry fasting, and new immune cells are created. Leading biogerontologist Valter Longo, director of the University of Southern California Longevity Institute, who has been lauded for his advancements in longevity research, has been finding similar results in his fasting-mimicking diets. Longo has proven that caloric restriction in conjunction with chemotherapy has tremendous effects on cancer patients. His studies have shown, like Dr. Filonov's, that fasting triggers stem cell regeneration and protects against immune system damage; the latter typically affects chemotherapy patients. In an interview, Dr. Longo explains that in his human and animal work, he noticed that the white blood cell count is reduced after a prolonged fast, but that during the rehydration and refueling period, the white blood cells come back.[3]

I venture that nothing can compare with the advanced autophagy that dry fasting ignites. Even consuming a small quantity of amino acids, or leucines, prevents autophagy from kicking in, so the fasting-mimicking diet, or intermittent fasting, cannot reproduce the effects of dry fasting.

As Dr. Filonov explains, cells get comfortable with incoming food and water and lose the ability to self-renew, as they get "lazy." Once the flow of food and water stops, old biomolecules die and decompose. "The body begins to take water from the air; therefore, the air must be very pure. Cells in our body begin to produce their own high-quality water from their internal reserves."

Over several consecutive days without food and water, cells fulfill their mission of finding alien material and destroying it. Normally, phagocytic cells are migrating around the body looking for prey in the form of fat that we eat. Instead of killing off diseased cells, they get distracted and consume fat from our foods. After being deprived of food and water for several consecutive days, however, the phagocytes fulfill their direct duties by seizing and digesting bacteria, cancer cells, viruses, and old dying cells. All pathologically altered tissues are fair game for the phagocytes.

Meanwhile, a powerful army of B-lymphocytes mobilizes from the gastrointestinal area, especially in the small intestines. The B-lymphocytes suppress and neutralize all existing pathogenic and alien elements, such as infections and parasites that almost never succumb to modern antibacterial therapy. During dry fasting, these pathogens are in turn destroyed by phagocytes and enzymes, which are activated by a state of acidosis that occurs by the eighth or ninth day without water.

Nine-day dry fasts increase red blood cells, white blood cells, hemoglobin, and platelets. Lymphocytes and monocytes increase in the blood by nearly 80 percent. As Dr. Filonov explained to me, "Since the body is not spending energy digesting food, the immune system cells—having received a powerful energy supply from red blood cells—cleanse tissues so that patients can recover from all manner of illnesses."

Myths Surrounding Dry Fasting

Since there has been limited access to Dr. Filonov's scientific research and clinical experience on dry fasting in English, many myths have been circulating about dry fasting, and most literature on the subject is spurious and ill informed. Outside of Dr. Filonov's work, I've found no reliable source that delineates the science of dry fasting.

I can dispel the myth that the body cannot exist for more than three days without water. One kilo of fat in the body can provide nourishment for the cells for two to three days alone, and I have watched both thin and obese patients dry fast for nine- to eleven-day periods successfully in Siberia under Dr. Filonov's supervision. Dry fasting does not cause kidney failure, electrolyte imbalances, or—worse—death.

The popular health psychic Anthony William, who does not have any medical training, writes bestselling books on healing with fruits and celery juice, among other plant-based formulas. He posted on

Instagram and on his popular blog that one should never dry fast: "Here's what you need to know about dry fasting: Never do it. Ever. This is traumatizing and harmful to your body and brain. It fills your bloodstream with so many poisons you can nearly go into sepsis. The toxins spill out of the liver but they don't get flushed out of the body. Dry fasting is incredibly destructive for your liver, kidneys, nervous system, and brain—it actually kills brain cells."[4]

William has obviously never dry fasted and does not understand the science behind it. If wild animals dry fast to survive, and if I dry fasted and came out feeling better than I ever have in my life, with a full recovery of my memory, which enabled me to speed-write two books within a year, then I really don't think I have killed off too many brain cells.

Dr. Filonov sternly says, "To criticize dry fasting, and to reject it, we must first of all be competent in this area." Having witnessed over a hundred patients dry fast for nine days at Dr. Filonov's clinic, I can report that patients are vivacious and healthy when they exit their fasts. People should not write about things they don't know about and haven't experienced.

Dry fasting does just the opposite of what Anthony William forecasts. Dr. Filonov writes that the kidneys and liver are on almost total rest. The brain is protected. "In the process of dry fasting, many organs and systems get physiological rest, which allows them to recover their damaged structures and functions," he explains.[5]

A Variety of Ailments Dry Fasting May Relieve

Dr. Filonov has treated a multiplicity of diseases with dry fasting. Regular, systematic dry fasting helps prevent cancer cells from forming. Dry fasting is a "major preventative measure against malignant tumors," according to Dr. Filonov. Dr. Filonov has treated numerous gynecological disorders, including infertility, ovarian cysts, uterine fibroids, and endometriosis. He has treated rheumatoid arthritis, bronchial asthma, hypertension, neurological diseases, chronic gastritis, and skin diseases including eczema and psoriasis.

He advises against dry fasting if one is severely underweight, lactating, pregnant, or has a history of disordered eating. In the case of elderly patients, he writes a specific protocol for each case but does not recommend extended dry fasts. If there are any other concerns about what condition may not tolerate dry fasting, I recommend taking these questions up directly with Dr. Filonov. (You can find his contact information on his website, which is given at the end of this chapter.) I can attest to the power of dry fasting to cure autoimmune disorders and even the most advanced cases of Lyme disease.

I have introduced dry fasting to four people from Europe and America who have reported back, "Michelle, I'm so grateful I found you," "My health is transforming," and "I owe you my life." The elegance of the dry fast is that it is free, and one can conduct it on one's own after having passed through the training.

Dr. Filonov writes that "fasting creates a second birth in the body," but little did he know how true this would be for me.[6] Dry fasting reincarnated me in the same body, so to maintain my second birth, I systematically dry fast on a regular basis. This prevents me from contracting illnesses or falling back into a state of ill health.

Although my genetic profile states that I'm missing certain detoxification enzymes, and the director of the European laboratory I visited wrote on my final report that the patient would need lifelong support to detoxify, Dr. Filonov reassures me that genetics are only 20 percent of an accurate health profile. The remaining 80 percent derives from lifestyle choices including diet, exercise, and systematic dry fasting.

This topic came up between us again when I submitted a saliva sample to 23andMe and discovered that I tested positive for ApoE4, the genetic variant for Alzheimer's disease.

Reading Dr. Dale Bredeson's groundbreaking work on reversing Alzheimer's, *The End of Alzheimer's: The First Program to Prevent and Reverse Cognitive Decline*, I learned that in addition to genetic variants, risk factors that contribute to Alzheimer's include Lyme disease, because the chronic inflammation that ensues in the aftermath of a tick bite causes cognitive decline.[7] Dr. Bredeson enumerates methylation deficiencies, high heavy-metal levels, chronic sinus issues, mold exposure, and amalgam fillings in his list of factors contributing to Alzheimer's. Many of the chronic Lyme patients I know also suffer from these ailments, but there's no need for alarm, thanks to the effective solution of dry fasting.

Those of us who suffer from chronic mysterious illnesses obsess about tests and lab results after years of perpetually seeking cures. Dr. Filonov set many of my inner fears to rest during the summer of 2018, when I returned to Siberia for a maintenance dry fast. When I lamented to him about the genetic variant I carried for Alzheimer's, he shook his wise head at me, and said that dry fasting would always protect me from Alzheimer's. "Michelle, dry fasting can remove the amyloid plaque found in the brains of patients with Alzheimer's. Your brain will not accumulate this abnormal protein since you systematically dry fast." This is coming from a practitioner who treated radiation patients from Chernobyl. He said that scientists in Russia have been proving that dry fasting can alter genetic variants. This information may prove invaluable and comforting to the striking percentage of chronic Lyme patients who also carry the genetic variant ApoE4 for Alzheimer's.

Dr. Filonov isn't the only one to promise protection from Alzheimer's through fasting. In the United States, Dr. Mattson's neuroscience lab found that in his animal subjects, alternate-day water fasting protects the brain. Like Dr. Filonov, Dr. Mattson reassures us that "nerve cells possess an innate ability to respond adaptively to intermittent dietary challenges in ways that help them perform better and counteract the adversities of aging, thereby potentially delaying the development of neurodegenerative diseases of aging like Alzheimer's and Parkinson's."[8] Dr. Mattson concludes that if people exercise frequently, reduce their caloric intake, and challenge their brains with intellectual challenges, they are far less likely to suffer from Alzheimer's, Parkinson's, or stroke.

What's been shown is that, when deprived of food, brain neurons launch a molecular defense against free radicals and pernicious amyloid plaque. Fasting promotes the growth of new neurons and increases the number of mitochondria in neurons; these strengthened connections between neurons increase one's ability to learn and enhance memory. Can you imagine what the brain can accomplish in this regard when challenged to a nine- or eleven-day dry fast? I would like to submit my own brain for testing at Dr. Mattson's laboratory.

My process of autophagy is not going to break down again; my body will clear its cellular detritus each time that I dry fast. I choose the scientific path of dry fasting as my internal, invisible fountain of youth, advanced by Nobel Prize–winning scientists, practiced for decades in Russia, and perfected by Dr. Filonov, and I will never look back.

• • •

Dr. Filonov conducts dry fasts regularly in his Siberian outpost and in various locations throughout Europe. For further information, you may consult his website: www.filonov.net.

18

A GUIDE TO DRY FASTING

One of the marvels of the world is the sight of a
soul sitting in prison with the key in its hand.

—Rumi, "The Sight of a Soul"

I offer a humble disclaimer as a prelude to this vital chapter. I'm not a certified nutritionist; nor am I a medical doctor. What I am is a Johns Hopkins–trained researcher who has confidence in my encyclopedic knowledge on the dry-fasting protocol and plant-based nutrition, based on my empirical research. I've followed Dr. Filonov's strict protocol for five years, and I have been in close contact with him. I've successfully dry fasted multiple times for periods of nine to eleven days. I have coached people with chronic illnesses through extended dry fasts. I will arm you with the requisite tools so that, should you choose, you can embark on your healing journey to clear the cellular detritus that clutters your path to rejuvenation.

Friends and strangers implore me to coach them through lengthy water fasts and dry fasts. I haven't had a single hiccup while coaching others through fasts; it comes naturally to me after years of trial and error in my own body. Although I had no way of knowing it at the time, all these practices were preparing me for my dry-fasting journey.

Fine-tuning the dry-fasting protocol has been the most arduous task of all. The human body does not remain static. I've practiced seasonally based eating for decades, so my food choices are frequently contingent on what organic fruits and vegetables are available to me locally. I share my kitchen tools, grocery lists, and recipes with you in Appendix C. I encourage you to improvise and create your own recipes. Although the protocol's many steps may seem draconian, they're in place for your safety. As Dr. Filonov cautions, "Dry fasting—in my experience—is the most effective kind of fasting, but if it is not properly prepared for and practiced, it is fraught with serious complications."[1] All the people I've coached have found that the protocol is easy to understand and follow. You will have unique needs based on your body's terrain. The terrain, or *milieu*, as French scientist Claude Bernard referred to it, is the internal ecosystem of the body, composed of over one trillion cells, and as my former naturopath in New York City, Dr. Anthony Salzarulo, explains it, if the terrain is out of whack, you are going to have symptoms. (He is my former naturopath only because I haven't needed a doctor since I went to Siberia.)

I've always cared deeply for the state of my body, mind, and spirit. I experimented incessantly with foods, quantities, and exercise to arrive at what I call a state of shining and bouncing.

Shining and bouncing is my ideal; it's my new normal, and I posit that every human can achieve it if I can. Dr. Filonov predicted that I would "fly" after dry fasting, but to do so, I make careful choices. I've systematically developed a dry-fasting protocol based on Dr. Filonov's exit lectures and my own dietary experiments. As Dr. Filonov's first American patient, who happens to be fastidious about notetaking, I share his wisdom with you, dear reader.

After I discovered Dr. Filonov that auspicious Saturday afternoon in bed, I attempted to research dry fasting further, yet all the information published in print and on the internet is spurious. Even those who advocate for dry fasting on the internet do not seem to have any experience in extended dry fasting; nor do they have a fraction of Dr. Filonov's medical background and training. In my protocol suggestions, I adhere to Dr. Filonov's medical dry-fasting system, and when I offer my own suggestions and interpretations, they're based on my successful experiences dry fasting.

Please take heed of Dr. Filonov's words that dry fasting can be fraught with serious complications if it isn't practiced according to a highly specific protocol. Dry fasting is not akin to green juice fasting, which Dr. Filonov calls a diet as opposed to a fast, and it's not even like water fasting. Although I started dry fasting cold turkey on a Saturday afternoon in my bed out of despair, I don't recommend that you drop whatever you're drinking right now and leap into it. Learn to dry fast with patience, dedication, and respect for the protocol.

When it comes to embarking on the dry-fasting journey, Rumi writes it best in his poem "Response to Your Question": "You may as well free a few words / from your vocabulary: *why* and *how* and *impossible.* / Open the mouth-cage and let those fly away."[2] The word "impossible" simply does not apply to dry fasting. Dry fasting is for all of us humans; it's not just for those who are deathly ill. I've heard Dr. Filonov say sadly that he wished people would come to him when they were healthy so that he could help them develop a practice of dry fasting for prevention.

My college friend Tats was so impressed with my successes when she visited me at Dr. Filonov's pop-up dry-fasting clinic in Kaliningrad in 2018, that she now water fasts two days a week, and consults with Dr. Filonov when he comes to Moscow. As Dr. Filonov has noted, "The older the body is, the less there is a chance of restoring youth. Fasting is extremely important for younger people as a means of reversing the aging process," so start as soon as possible.

Preparing the Mind for Fasting

So, how does one begin? The body works hard during dry fasting, but if the mind is stressed, the body cannot do its work effectively. If the spirit is not at peace, the mind acts up, and it may desire unhealthy substances, including alcohol, drugs, or nicotine. All these substances should be tapered off and eliminated in preparation for the fast. In tandem, stress-relieving techniques such as meditation should be incorporated daily. Therefore, before the body can embark on its work, one has to cleanse one's mind and spirit.

This is a three-pronged protocol, encompassing body, mind, and spirit. Each prong is critical. The body is the doctor, doing the work of dry fasting, but the mind and spirit have equally important roles. The mind should rest. Fasting and spirituality are inextricably linked; it's nearly impossible to fast without experiencing a heightened spiritual awareness. It's no accident, as Dr. Filonov notes, that the Old Testament mentions fasting seventy-five times. Moses fasted for forty days, purportedly without food or water, so that his face was shining rays once he exited. Having experienced this shining effect after merely ten days of fasting without food or water, this is not implausible to me. Mohammed, Buddha, and Jesus fasted for the quintessential forty-day period as a spiritual rite of passage into higher-order spiritual leadership.

Dr. Filonov notes that the ancient Persian sun worshippers, Celtic Druids, and Ancient Egyptian priests conducted long periods of dry fasting as an initiation into the higher realms of spirituality. Dr. Filonov points out that we find fragments of writing on dry fasting as a spiritual tool in Tibet, Greece, Persia, India, Scandinavia, China, Rome, and Egypt. In North America, young Native American warriors in training were left on mountaintops for four days and four nights to dry fast without food and water. These dry fasts were rites of passage meant to purify and strengthen the men, thereby creating the physical, mental, and spiritual fortitude required to be a warrior.

Like the young warriors, it's essential to be in a good place psychologically and spiritually before you start dry fasting. The body cannot do its work effectively if there are deep-seated habits of emotional overeating that will creep back in during the exit. If you find yourself perennially hungry, unsatisfied by food, but always eating, ask yourself what you are hungry for. What is it that you are trying to fill yourself up with? Are you hungry for love, approval, security, or comfort? Try to find healthy ways to fill yourself up, like taking walks in the park, spending time with friends and animals, or finding an artistic outlet for your worries. Overeating will never satisfy an emotional void, and it will contribute to the inflammation that fuels chronic illness.

Stress also affects the body adversely. Consider how you can mitigate worries and anxieties before you fast. Even if you cannot change your circumstances, you can rely on breathing exercises, meditation, and yoga to alleviate stress. Dr. Filonov recommends using pranic yogic breathing to oxygenate the cells before, during, and after fasting.

Leading trauma scientist Bessel van der Kolk foregrounds the role of the body in healing from trauma in his revolutionary book *The Body Keeps the Score*. His research shows that the body retains cellular memories of past trauma, or, as the idiomatic expression goes, "The issues are in the tissues." As you embark on the dry-fasting journey, the issues will come out of the tissues, and it's best to do some psychological preparation for this shift either on your own or with the help of a therapist.

Psychological preparation for dry fasting involves shedding the identity of being a chronically ill person and embracing the possibility of being fully recovered and healthy. Referring to oneself as a "lymie" or a "moldie" concretizes one's identity as a sick person. When you call yourself a "lymie," you allow the disease to metastasize from the physical body to infiltrate the mind and spirit so that you are your disease. I had hidden behind my illness for so long that I identified as an invalid rather than as a viable individual.

Virginia Woolf writes, "In illness . . . we cease to be soldiers in the army of the upright. We become deserters."[3] I was used to being a deserter, and I had copped out on many things as a result: "No, I haven't finished turning my dissertation into a book because I have been ill. No, I don't run marathons anymore." I had become used to feeling unworthy and sitting on the sideline of functioning society, invisible. I had to shed that mantra: "I'm sick, so I can't." Let go of the sick persona. You cannot be well while repeating the "I am sick" mantra.

The inner voices that the chronically ill use to speak to themselves are frequently not kind and should be softened before one embarks on the dry-fasting journey. I was self-critical for decades until I became bedridden with Lyme. Pay attention to your inner voice. Are you kind to yourself when no one is listening but you? The chronically ill patients I've encountered have a historically hard time loving themselves. It's time to shed this judgment.

Cultivate an inner voice that is kind, positive, and encouraging, rather than critical and negative. Self-compassion will go a long way in contributing to your healing. While you are dry fasting, gently ask your mind to take a break so the body can focus on its work. I do this by releasing any anxious thoughts and focusing on calming breaths. I've included a section of meditations at the back of this book for you to consult as needed.

Preparing the Body

Once you've prepared your mind and spirit for their roles, you can turn your attention to the physical body. The doctor is ready to begin its work and you will need to assist. Try to think of the process as fasting pioneer Herbert Shelton describes it: "Fasting is a rest—a physiological vacation. It is not an ordeal nor a penance. It is a house-cleaning measure which deserves to be better known and more widely used."[4] Work with your body to facilitate the "house cleaning."

First, stop taking all supplements and vitamins and any medications that are not vital. On the days that you dry fast, take no medications at all. For questions about the use of medications, I recommend writing to Dr. Filonov. (His website is provided at the end of Chapter 17.) I've seen several patients who no longer needed medications after dry fasting, but I cannot counsel anyone in this regard.

Lyme patients tend to take a staggering number of supplements. I was taking twenty-five or more tablets a day when I stopped cold turkey to begin Dr. Filonov's protocol. Researchers at the Friedrich Schiller University Jena in Germany found that supplements inhibit the body's natural stress response,[5] so don't be alarmed by the prospect of going off supplements. If they worked, you wouldn't be contemplating dry fasting.

These are the steps that Dr. Filonov asked me to take before I arrived in Siberia. If you become Dr. Filonov's patient, he will provide you with a personalized protocol. For two weeks before embarking on the first dry fast, take two tablets of activated charcoal on an empty stomach either in the morning or in the evening. Upon waking, have one teaspoon of aluminum-free baking soda in an eight-ounce cup of hot water each day for two weeks. Increase your water intake to at least two liters per day of high-quality spring or filtered water—no tap water that is chlorinated.

I cannot underscore this enough: dry fasting will not feel good unless you do proper spring cleaning on your physical home to the best of your ability. You may do dry skin brushing, far infrared saunas, cryotherapy, colonics, or any cleansing rituals that you may already have in place. One Ayurvedic practice that I recommend is called oil pulling. It involves swirling a tablespoon of coconut oil in your mouth in the morning for one minute and spitting it out before brushing your teeth. You may exfoliate dry skin and stimulate circulation with a body brush using circular strokes, which is called dry brushing.

These treatments will not cure you, but they will ease detox symptoms that you might experience on the first fasts. The more you cleanse your body in advance, the easier it is to dry fast.

In preparation for the dry fast, avoid harsh chemicals from housecleaning agents, nail polish and remover, and chemical makeup. Try to use only organic, nontoxic products. If you don't have nontoxic lotion, you can use organic coconut oil on your face and hands and as a body lotion. I trashed all my products that weren't organic and discovered RMS makeup and Tata Harper facial products.

When I was in the throes of chronic Lyme, I would ask my doctors in the States what I should be eating for a healthy anti-Lyme diet. They said that diet represented 2 percent of the Lyme problem. I disagreed then, and I disagree even more vehemently after dry fasting. The quality and quantity of what you eat determines how you feel.

The body can't be happy getting plugged with junk every day, or even with excessive amounts of organic food.

Eliminate any sugar, processed foods, fast foods, junk food, and snacks from your diet. When you feel confident with these new practices, avoid heavy meat-based meals and simple starches. I veer from gluten and dairy. Gravitate toward low-glycemic berries for breakfast, light salads for lunch, and steamed vegetables with wild-caught, low-mercury fish like salmon or cod for dinner. Try to purchase organic produce as much as possible. Wean yourself from caffeine and alcohol and choose herbal teas instead. Favor whole-grain hot cereals like millet or buckwheat kasha, as opposed to bread or processed cereals. In Appendix C, I include sample grocery lists and a variety of nutrient-dense recipes to guide you.

As you prepare for the fasting, begin to reduce your caloric load. Pay attention to your portions. Do you feel full after meals? If so, can you reduce the portions so that you are practicing caloric restriction as a first step toward fasting? You may use intermittent fasting to ease into the fasting process, by maintaining an eating window that is eight to twelve hours long to allow your body time for digestion and rest between meals. Savoring smaller meals before fasting makes the transition far easier. It's less of a shock if we allow the body a chance to taper from food to dry fasting. You may nourish the body during this cleansing period with homemade vegetable broths, freshly pressed vegetables juices, and any of the recipes I share from my own protocol in Appendix C.

If it's possible—and it may not be for patients with chronic illnesses—practice taking long, slow walks in nature, and incorporate gentle stretching or yoga into your daily routine. Because of my weakened state, it wasn't possible for me to take daily walks in preparation, so be gentle with yourself as you do what you can.

It was too late for me to learn the lesson that Dr. Filonov teaches his patients as an introduction to dry fasting: "Do not dry fast without attempting to water fast first." I even recommend green juice fasting for a few days before one starts water fasting. Dr. Filonov thinks that juice fasting floods the body with too much glucose, but if one juices vegetables like romaine lettuce, celery, kale, parsley, and lemon, then the concoctions are low-glycemic. I've included juicing recipes in Appendix C.

On the day before your first water or dry fast, only drink liquids, beginning with fresh-squeezed lemon juice in warm water upon waking. Dr. Filonov and many others advocate for doing this each morning. Follow this with a fresh-squeezed vegetable juice or a pureed vegetable soup for lunch, and perhaps conclude the day with a homemade vegetable broth for dinner.

The shorter twenty-four-hour and three-day water and dry fasts can be conducted nearly anywhere. Based on Dr. Filonov's advice and my experience, a seven- or nine-day dry fast should only take place in nature, preferably in the mountains near streams. The body will absorb any pollution in the air while dry fasting, and the environment must be very pure. I have dry fasted in the Berkshire hills of Massachusetts, in Manhattan, and on the polluted streets of Houston. There is a notable difference. Find a quiet and comforting spot where you will be surrounded by both nature and positive energy.

As Dr. Filonov underscores in his first book, "It is extraordinarily important that dry fasting takes place in a favorable psychological climate."[6] Seek the company of people who support your healing journey. Do not discuss the fast with those who respond negatively to this form of healing. These steps are critical, for one becomes very sensitive while dry fasting. The body is healing, and additional emotional stress will undermine the delicate process. Although I find dry fasting to be a solitary practice, and one that brings much peace and contemplation, the times I've dry fasted with a friend have brought solace, too.

In the winter of 2018, Isabella, an Italian patient suffering from chronic Epstein-Barr, came to Kaliningrad with me to Dr. Filonov's pop-up clinic on the banks of the icy Baltic Sea. She had been bedridden on and off for years. She was eager to try the method that healed me; this year she was out skiing again on the Italian slopes, and we just had a celebratory reunion in Rome to toast our renewed health. Isabella and I shared a *dacha* in the countryside outside Kaliningrad, and we took long walks along the snowy banks of the Baltic by the pastel light of the sky. It was deeply comforting to dry fast together, and we even enjoyed excursions into Kaliningrad to see Kant's tomb and hear a sublime organ recital; music does nourish the soul while one is dry fasting. If you do have a friend with whom you can fast, and if you're skittish at all about dry fasting, the solidarity could prove helpful.

Refrain from broadcasting your dry fast on social media or to your friends and family. Hearing "but you are going to die" from people who have no experience with dry fasting will not boost your morale. My positive reinforcement from D, Dad, and Janet brought me immeasurable strength while I was dry fasting, but I strategically chose that inner circle of support.

It's counterproductive to be in a dry, indoor environment, particularly in the winter. When I was dry fasting in Kaliningrad last winter, there was no space to sleep outside, and the *dacha* was heated with electric baseboards, which dried me out terribly. I wrote on my day seven, "My mouth is caked and cracked like a desert floor. I worry about choking on my tongue." If you can dry fast and be outdoors to absorb the dew in the air, that's ideal. Or keep the windows open at night; try to avoid environments like the one I had in Kaliningrad.

To water fast, after conducting the careful preparation and tapering your food intake, choose a designated day, and consume water only from the time you wake up until the following morning. Ease into eating again with a piece of fruit for breakfast, with the exception of citrus, followed by a finely chopped salad for lunch and dinner. Chart how your body feels on a one-day water fast, pause for a few days, and then continue on to a three-day water fast. Pause for as long as a week, and water fast for seven days. I have seen several patients who had no time to prepare and jumped right into a dry fast without water fasting, but Dr. Filonov recommends preparing with water fasts first.

On the evening before your dry fast, take a shower and use coconut oil to hydrate your body. You may practice the soothing Ayurvedic oil massage called self-abhyanga by warming a quarter cup of coconut oil, or oil of your choice, and spreading it over your entire body. Dress in loose, comfortable clothing, preferably with natural fibers.

During the Fast

Your first twenty-four-hour dry fast will begin when you go to sleep in the evening, so it's slightly longer than twenty-four hours. If you begin on a Friday night, then you will not consume anything until Sunday morning when you wake up.

Remember that you will not have any contact with any substances while you are training to dry fast, so there will be no brushing of the teeth, showering, or applying lip balm and lotion. It would be dangerous and counterproductive to administer enemas or colonics while dry fasting. As Dr. Filonov says, "This is necessary to prevent cells from coming in contact with water and interrupting the autophagy process." Dr. Filonov says one day of dry fasting is more effective for clearing cellular detritus than three days of water fasting.

While you're training your body to dry fast for extended periods, you may incorporate cold-water therapy through ice baths, ice-cold showers, or dunking in icy rivers. After you have successfully passed through a nine-day dry fast, you may break the fast with cold-water therapy. That means that you can take an ice-cold shower on the designated weekly day that you dry fast. Dutch expert Wim Hof has shown how cold-water therapy combined with breathing exercises can repress the inflammatory response in the body.[7]

Aim to spend time in nature. Walk for up to ten kilometers, or six miles, on your dry-fasting days at a slow and deliberate pace, which will accelerate fat-burning mechanisms. Dr. Filonov encourages walking as much as possible; he explains that it facilitates autophagy and assists in clearing cellular waste. Given that many readers may have chronic illnesses in which chronic fatigue is a primary symptom, please do not be alarmed if this is not possible. Even if you are walking slowly, gradually increase daily walks. Please do not engage in any rigorous exercise such as running or weightlifting, though.

Perhaps try a digital detox from email and the phone for the days that you're fasting, to rest your mind. I find that digital overstimulation is draining in today's hyper-plugged-in environment. A digital detox does wonders for recharging one's natural energy. Dry fasting prompted me to monitor my relationship with my addictive smart phone. It has been refreshing and energizing to spend time in person with friends and observe the natural world around me without being glued to my phone.

You may experience random aches, pains, headaches, or other symptoms, but don't be alarmed, as they all fall within the normal realm of dry fasting. They shift quickly. Headaches are common if one hasn't eliminated caffeine or alcohol well in advance of the dry fast. Fatigue can set in like a low fog. These symptoms do not mean that the mythologies of dry fasting are going to come true and your body is shutting down; it's merely a messy process to vacuum one's body of cellular decay.

The symptoms recede as one progressively trains the body to dry fast. To encourage you, I can share that I experienced virtually no symptoms on my last recent fast of eleven days—even my tongue looked pure and free from mucus on day eleven—and my exit was seamless. I was running at high speeds the day after I started eating solid foods again. Breathing through the symptoms meditatively will sustain you through the first dry fasts, as your body seizes the opportunity to chomp through diseased cells.

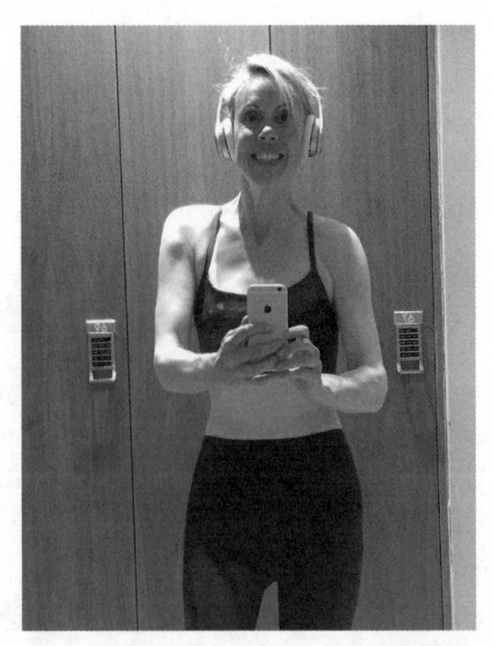

Back to running after an eleven-day dry fast in Siberia, spring 2019

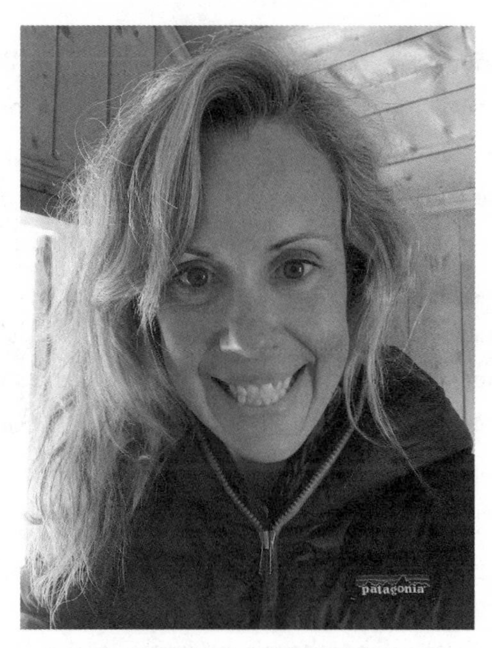

Lyme-free Miche in Siberia, 2019

I guide myself through visual meditations to accompany the intangible healing work taking place inside my body. I imagine that I am breathing in healing light that spreads through my body, eradicating compromised cells. As I exhale, I imagine that compromised cells are leaving my body. I used to say silently to my body, "Lyme is not welcome here. Candida and psoriasis are not welcome here. Vibrant cells: grow stronger."

My mantra in Siberia was "The body is the doctor—it is healing. The mind can go free and rest while the body does its work. Spirit is holding space for all of this healing work." I kept visualizing this, and I believed it to be true. This mantra is meant to be shared, since it was powerful for me.

Spiritual epiphanies bubble into my thoughts while I dry fast, prompting me to feel as if I have a direct line to the etheric realm; I thought it might be because I had meditated for so many years. Thus,

I didn't mention it to the Lyme, mold, and Epstein-Barr patients I coached this year. I created individualized protocols for them before they embarked on lengthy dry fasts, but I didn't think to mention, "Oh, by the way, you might have a spiritual awakening during the dry fasting." To my astonishment, every one of them came to me in awe of the spiritual experiences they had. They would ask tentatively, "Is there a spiritual side to this?" The resounding answer is yes. Working in conjunction with one another, the body, mind, and spirit incinerate anxiety and stress, just as they destroy diseased cells. While you are literally starving, spiritual nutrition feeds you and strengthens your resolve.

If you feel faint at heart, or if you're tempted by the allure of water, resist. If you can endure the suffering generated by the vicissitudes of chronic Lyme disease—or, insert any diseases from cancer to autoimmune diseases and chronic mystery illnesses here—then you can endure a dry fast. Your motivation will be high, generated by the despair of being faced with unacceptable sensations that are the antithesis of normal.

Do not out of desperation try rinsing your mouth with water. It will only make it drier, and it will be harder to continue the dry fast, given the amplified thirst. Furthermore, it will interrupt the radical autophagy taking place as your body clears out diseased cells, because you'll be providing fuel to your body.

Sleeping may be difficult as you acclimate to dry fasting, and if that's the case for you, try napping during the day when you feel tired and resting with your eyes closed at night. The meditative breathing helps with sleeping in a majority of cases, but sleep may be elusive for some. Furthermore, the body reacts differently with each successive dry fast, so sleep may come easier as your body adapts.

Congratulate yourself and your body for beginning the training process for radical autophagy.

Exiting the Fast

When you wake on Sunday morning of your twenty-four-hour dry fast, for example, you will break your fast. Take a cold shower. Then prepare a hot thermos of tea-temperature spring water. Do not use any chlorinated water; Dr. Filonov argues that this acts as a poison in the body. Mountain Valley spring water in glass bottles is ideal but use the best water available to you. It's quite important to only drink hot water after you break a dry fast. Since your internal temperature is higher as your body burns cellular debris, it's a shock to the body to drink cold water.

During the first few exits, it's comforting to have someone tend to you, but if that's not possible, just take extra care with yourself. If you're feeling weak and tired the first days, please rest as much as your body requests. Do not expect miraculous results from the first dry fasts. They are preliminary.

Dr. Filonov recommends conducting a twenty-four-hour dry fast several times before continuing on to a three-day fast. I didn't have the luxury of time to do this. In the case of an accelerated treatment plan in the face of dire illness, pause for at least one week between the twenty-four-hour and the three-day dry fast. Follow the twenty-four-hour protocol for the three-day fast.

Fasting is a destroyer, as Dr. Filonov tells his patients during the exit lectures. By contrast, the exit builds up the body. Short fasts do not require much building up, as there is still much detritus to destroy in the body until one has completed a series of nine-day dry fasts. After twenty-four hours of dry fasting, Dr. Filonov says that human growth hormone gets released, which produces a rejuvenating effect. Although dry fasting stimulates the metabolism during the exit period, use caution not to overeat after one-day fasts. The objective is not to seesaw in a fasting-feasting cycle but rather to modulate from fasting to caloric restriction while training for extended dry fasts.

The exit is critical, for, as Dr. Filonov explains, "it holds 70 percent of the therapeutic value; it must be conducted perfectly." I repeat these imperative words later in this chapter. The fast is not over when you start drinking. That's when the hard work happens as you navigate the mine field of food choices and quantities that are available to you. The body will take back calories very quickly, since it's been in a deprived state. I brought a wooden bowl back from Siberia that fits no more than one and a half cups of food, and I strictly eat from that bowl during my exits.

After a one-day dry fast, after consuming hot water for the morning, you may have a piece of fresh fruit for lunch, and fresh vegetables for dinner if you're hungry. If hunger doesn't return, remain on liquids until it does. I can't shock my body with solid food—rather, I taper slowly. Remain on a plant-based diet to continue cleansing, especially if you're preparing for longer dry fasts.

On the second day after you exit, you may have a small portion of millet or buckwheat kasha for breakfast, vegetable soup for lunch with no salt or oil, and salad with no dressing for dinner. "If a person only eats plant foods, the effect of starvation continues during the meals," Dr. Filonov explains.

If you choose to follow the Siberian exit diet, you'll consume a small portion of porridge for breakfast with fruit, a salad for lunch, and a soup or steamed vegetable with fish soup for dinner. Then you may experiment—your body will tell you if you choose foods poorly or if you consume too much.

Some of the people with Lyme I've coached through dry fasting have expressed to me that they can't tolerate nightshade vegetables, lectins, and fruit. One said, "But Michelle, I cannot do lectins." Another said, "Michelle, I'll bloat up like a blimp if I eat watermelon."

I assure them that as their terrain changes in response to dry fasting, their bodies will tolerate foods heretofore *verboten.* They have all reported back that this was true. "How can it be? Maybe I should become a fruitarian," one patient wrote back after he went from being a frequent meat eater to craving nothing but watermelon after his successful nine-day dry fast to beat Lyme.

When you start eating after a dry fast, chew every bite of food until it is pulverized into juice-like pureed form before you swallow it. Therapeutic chewing predigests food, assisting in the laborious digestion process. Multiple studies have proven that it also facilitates weight loss, although it may not contribute to your social standing at dinners, sadly. Allow at least four hours between meals to prevent food from fermenting in the digestive tract. Otherwise, you may experience gas and bloating.

If you experience any nausea or unpleasant symptoms during the exit, these are all normal reactions to the radical process of accelerated autophagy. Take two tablets of activated charcoal and one teaspoon of aluminum-free baking soda stirred in hot water. If your stomach bothers you from overeating, or if you've chosen foods that resonated poorly with your body, return to drinking water only until bloating and gas subside.

In the first two to three weeks after fasting, depending on the length of the fast, exclude alcohol, caffeine, spicy foods, fat, canned food, smoked food, salt, and oil. If you are going to fractionally dry fast and increase your dry-fasting days incrementally, then stay on the exit diet of fruit, vegetables, whole grains, and fish throughout the fasting and exiting periods. After a nine-day fast, abstain from meat for one month, and sugar is discouraged for the long term.

Dr. Filonov recommends consuming thirty milliliters of water per kilogram of body weight. Above all, Dr. Filonov insists that the water be as pure as possible. Most of the post-dry-fasting problems such as constipation arise because the patient hasn't consumed enough water. A simple way to test hydration levels, he says, is by checking the urine stream to see if it is pale yellow—dark yellow indicates dehydration. Since 70 percent of the human body is composed of water, we must nourish our bodies adequately with this life force energy that we'll appreciate more than ever after dry fasting.

Longer Dry Fasts

As you embark on longer dry fasts, envision what your dream life will be like once you are rejuvenated in body, mind, and spirit. You could write out qualities that you associate with yourself but may have lost sight of in the face of chronic illness. Create a vision board on a large poster and write out the projects you dream of realizing, from "creating renewable energy products," to "volunteering," to "writing a screenplay." This is powerful work, and it helps manifest a new life post–dry fasting.

To continue what I call the marathon-training program for dry fasting, you may fractionally train up to the extended seven-day dry fast. There are a number of ways to do this. On Dr. Filonov's fractional program, you would dry fast for one day, take one day off, then dry fast for two days. You would then exit for two days and then embark on a three-day dry fast. Next, you would exit for three days, launch into a four-day dry fast, exit for four days, and dry fast for five days. Alternatively, you may exit for a week in between fasts, so that you progress from a one-day to a three-day with a week-long exit interval, followed by a five-day dry fast and yet another week to exit before leaping into a seven-day dry fast.

While you're dry fasting for longer periods, let the body do its work as you rest. The body goes into the first stage of acidosis during days two through four. Once the body has exhausted reserves of glucose, it begins to consume stored reserves and secondary tissues, activating phagocytes and enzymes. The second—and most critical—acidotic crisis lasts from approximately the fifth to eighth days of dry fasting. The acidotic crisis catapults the body into high gear as autophagy obliterates weak cells. "The most important thing is to pass through the acidotic crisis, for during this second period of autolysis, the host defenses activate forcefully, working to cure many diseases," Dr. Filonov counsels. The body starts to heat up through the second acidotic crisis. This happened to me on the seventh day of my dry fast in Kaliningrad, as I wrote, "I have to keep putting my metal battery pack on the windowsill at night, and when it is cold enough, I run it up and down my organs like my liver. My organs are heating up as they heal."

During the first lengthy dry fasts, a thick mucus will accumulate on the tongue in various shades of white, yellow, and green. You may take an Ayurvedic tongue scraper or a plain old spoon to scrape your tongue each day that you dry fast. The lips chap and flake, and the skin begins to glow in rosy hues. The activated ketone bodies fuel the growth of new amino acids, which leads to tissue regeneration. None of these occurrences should be cause for alarm.

One is going to experience multiple symptoms during the lengthy dry fasts, but it was the first short dry fasts that were the absolute worst for me. Then my body was at its most toxic state. To reiterate, headaches, rashes, swollen lymph nodes, sore throats, joint pain, nausea, weakness, and fatigue are all normal within the realm of dry fasting. They will pass, and they're just the result of the body cleansing itself. The blood pressure may drop, and the pulse may slow down a bit. The body is merely clearing at a rapid rate. Dry fasting is not like taking yet another pill to sweep the disease under the rug—the rug is being burned entirely, along with everything beneath it.

Although you'll not be able to replicate the treatments offered at Dr. Filonov's center, you can schedule cupping appointments at many acupuncture offices. You may find lotion-free dry massages to be therapeutic, for they release muscle aches and decongest tissues while you are dry fasting. Shiatsu massage is an excellent option, for one remains fully clothed in loose-fitted clothing.

At the end of a lengthy fast, such as a nine-day one, before I break the fast, I feel that I've been overhauled and rejuvenated. My step is light—if a bit weary—my smile is radiant, and I feel content. Other dry fasters report the same sensations.

There's a sharp difference between the sensation of dry fasting and the feelings of exhaustion during the exit. If you feel weak and tired after the five-day dry fast, know that it's only temporary and that, within a week or two, your immunity will be strengthened, and you'll feel energetic. Each exit is different, so it may take longer for some to feel their strength and health returning, but do not despair through the delicate exit period. Your body has just undergone natural surgery, and you must rest.

I cannot recommend attempting a nine-day dry fast at home—it should be conducted the first time under medical supervision. At this point, the only medically sound place in the world to undergo a nine-day dry fast is at Dr. Filonov's clinic in Siberia, or at one of his pop-up clinics in Slovenia, Bulgaria, Turkey, or Italy, which take place throughout the year. Dr. Filonov is cautious and doesn't recommend dry fasting for more than five days at home alone the first time without his supervision. Do not strategize to dry fast for inordinately long periods to eradicate all the diseased tissues. I have seen some accounts on social media sharing dry fasts of twenty days; this is extremely dangerous and should not ever be attempted. The pendulum between life and death swings in a delicate balance. The systematic plan I have provided suffices.

When you take your cold-water exit shower after a five- to nine-day dry fast, do not use any toothpaste or cosmetics right away. Just use water for the first shower and wait until you have hydrated your body throughout the day before using toothpaste or lotion.

Prepare a thermos of hot water, and slowly swirl it around your dry mouth to soften the tissue and break up any deposits of mucus on your tongue. Spit out the first few sips that are laced with mucus. After five days of dry fasting or more, stay on hot water for at least twenty-four hours before continuing the normal exit protocol I outline here and in Appendix B.

On the morning following your hot-water day, you may have watermelon for breakfast, but make sure that it's organic, as the pesticides in watermelon will be far more damaging to the body after it has been cleansed by dry fasting. Then follow the exit plan for the one-day fast, and use the grocery list and recipes outlined in Appendix C.

Exiting from an extended dry fast is not to be taken lightly—the first twenty-one days are a critical period of healing. The body is regenerating white blood cells and stem cells, and it's rather fragile. I felt far weaker during the first nine-day exit than I did during the dry fasting itself. After the second long dry fast, I was stronger during the exit. There's no homogenous dry fast. Just like each one of our terrains is unique, each dry fast cannot be predicted. I can give you guidelines, but your experience will be unique to you.

Dr. Filonov is vehement about the following dictum: "After exiting, the food must be perfect." I cannot underscore this enough. Dr. Filonov has observed countless exits in which symptoms return because patients abused their bodies and didn't respect the protocol. "Most people are constantly sick because they are trying to recycle a huge amount of excess food they absorb," he says. He recommends that "if you overeat at any time, dry fast for a day, and then follow a lighter protocol," but this should be avoided during the up-building phase following a lengthy dry fast.

Please do not intermittently fast during the up-building period of the exit; your body requires nourishment during this time, not more starvation. Do not follow any "keto" or "Paleo" protocols such as the intermittent-fasting protocol that allows pork bellies and heavy dairy items. Foods like pork bellies that I see in certain intermittent-fasting plans are devastating on the liver after a dry fast, and your body will communicate this loudly. An excess of protein in the body merely converts to glucose and then to fat, which contributes to the aging process.

In Siberia, Dr. Filonov includes an organic kefir in his exit protocol, one that provides the body with essential probiotics, but I'm skittish about consuming milk products that are intended to raise six-hundred-pound calves with casein proteins but are not necessarily synergistic with the human body.

You become very sensitive to food when you are dry fasting and exiting, so you can enjoy a new relationship with your body based on intuition. In my case, I do best with a mostly raw vegan diet with a little wild-caught salmon. When Dr. Filonov's previous cook tried to push grain on me, I couldn't linguistically express that it was the wrong fuel for my body. I like to explain my fueling needs with a car analogy. I wouldn't put diesel into a Porsche 911 high-performance engine that required premium octane gas, which would be the highest quality fuel for its performance needs. For me, eating a bowl of porridge for breakfast is like putting diesel in my body, whereas eating a bowl of watermelon, or drinking a large glass of fresh-squeezed celery, cucumber, lemon, and ginger juice for breakfast is like putting premium octane gas into my tank. Only then I can run and write, or, as Dr. Filonov predicted, *fly*.

The people with chronic Lyme and mold whom I've been coaching through dry fasting have all been very anxious to eat the right foods on the dry-fasting entrances and exits, and over the long term. They've asked me to type up a protocol with the exact quantities of the perfect foods to eat, but I do not have a magical map. It's an inherently heuristic process to discover one's unique nutritional ideal. That is, you have to discover what the optimum fuel is for your body by trial, error, and success. It's like choosing your own adventure, albeit a well-informed one.

The foods that will provide you with the proper fuel are individual to you and your distinctive terrain. In your gut, you have about a hundred trillion microbes that influence health, weight, and energy levels. They are uniquely formed by the experiences you've had since birth—including the kind of birth that you had. If I eat the same food that is perfect for you, I may experience bloating and indigestion, whereas you might be flooded with peak energy.

At the Weizman Institute of Science in Israel, scientists Dr. Eran Segal and Dr. Eran Elinav created the Personalized Nutrition Project, which tracked hundreds of volunteers who wore blood-sugar monitors and meticulously charted their minute reactions to each food and liquid they consumed, along with their sleeping and exercise habits. Dr. Segal and Dr. Elinav's findings showed that although the volunteers were all consuming the same foods, their reactions were wildly divergent. Some volunteers experienced dramatic rises in blood sugar in response to certain foods, while others were not affected at all by the same foods.[8] The Personalized Nutrition Project is evidence that no one person can provide you with a detailed chart of what you should eat on the dry-fasting lifestyle. I can share a generalized series of recommendations that include what I call largely innocuous foods.

Although Dr. Filonov's dry-fasting method far transcends the ascetic demands of a monk, his exit plan involves a few surprisingly hedonistic treats: "You may drink high-quality matcha green tea from Japan. When you get home, drink organic coffee because it is replete with antioxidants. You may drink high-quality dry red wine for its antioxidants and health-giving properties—start by having a half-cup of red wine in hot water." Dr. Filonov lauds the "polyphenols," or phytochemicals with antioxidants found in green tea, coffee, and extra virgin olive oil, which reduce inflammation. This doesn't mean that you have to consume these substances. They are stimulants, after all. I share them because they may cheer some readers who are daunted by the task of being so abstemious.

A Lifelong Commitment

Dry fasting is not a one-time event. It's a lifelong practice that involves not only diet but also exercise, as Dr. Filonov explains: "I recommend a high level of physical activity, along with a systematic program of dry fasting." Exercise is a critical component of the post-dry-fasting lifestyle. It took me two nine-day dry fasts before I was able to exercise intensively. Exercise is as individual as food is; thus, one body might thrive on walking and yoga, while yet another craves running and hiking. After I broke the eleven-day dry fast in Siberia I describe in the following chapter, I was back to running ten kilometers a day right after I started eating solid foods again—my body is healthy enough to do so now. The question as to what kind of movement your body needs can only be answered by you.

Short fasts, even successive ones, will never accomplish the radical autophagy that a nine-day or ten-day dry fast will achieve. The days must be successive without interruption, and above all *without* water intake. The body does more serious healing work the longer that you fast. On the eleven-day dry fast I just completed in Siberia a few weeks ago, Dr. Filonov told everyone that my eleventh day alone was accomplishing what would take fifteen days of water fasting to achieve.

Do not ever say in a defeatist way, "Oh, I tried that dry-fasting technique, and it didn't work for me." I echo Rumi when it comes to fighting off chronic diseases like Lyme: "Half-heartedness does not reach into majesty."[9] You have to train your body incrementally to dry fast. Fast twice for nine-day periods within two months before you come to such negative conclusions. I guarantee that once you undertake this colossal effort, you will not fall back on the old Lyme (or chronic disease) identity.

The gift of health is the fountain of youth within, and you can give it to yourself. The key to the prison cell of chronic disease is yours, and it's found in these pages. Persevere with dry fasting, and I predict that you will be reborn into a new body with a cleansed mind and spirit. Dear reader, I would like to be the first to wish you a happy new birthday when you become your superhuman self.

19

CRIMES AGAINST WISDOM

For those who have an intense urge for wisdom,
it sits near them, waiting.

–Patanjali, *The Yogic Sutras of Patanjali*

I walked out of Siberia and onto the plane bound for New York in October 2017 feeling invincible, energetic, and lighthearted—feelings I hoped would last forever. My discipline was strong in Siberia. My desire to survive propelled me to dry fast. Upon my return to Manhattan, eager to celebrate my rejuvenation with friends, I shared communion portions of wine and foodie meals sized just right for Goldilocks's baby bear.

D and I celebrated my return with our friend Asif at Craft, where I nibbled on a side of broccoli rabe massaged with garlic and olive oil. I snuck a few bites of autumnal root vegetables that had been roasted with extra virgin olive oil, one of my favorite flavors. D watched over me with widened eyes, admonishing me, "No, there's too much olive oil for you! Don't eat the vegetables!"

And he was right. Even that seemingly innocuous meal with oily vegetables caused my stomach to pipe up in protest. After that I dialed it back to steamed vegetables, chopped salads, and the fresh-squeezed vegetable juice from Juice Generation that I'd been craving the entire time I was in Siberia.

I navigated this first important exit quite well, and I wish I could write, "and I followed the ideal post-dry-fasting protocol from that point forth." But that's just not how this narrative goes.

Over the past three decades, I've read countless studies, articles, and books on equations for achieving longevity and health, but my attempts to put these theories into a sustainable practice have resulted in some foolhardy choices among the prudent ones, which I share here at the expense of my dignity. The following embarrassing stories illustrate my bumpy journey to reach a synthesis between feasting and fasting. Dry fasting eradicated all traces of my chronic illness and left me with the most vivacious version of myself, and I have sought to maintain that quasi-superhuman place. But the first year and a half was like settling the wild west in my body. I urge you to learn from my mistakes rather than recreating them.

A couple of years after my first Siberian trip, I was at Kripalu studying in an intensive yoga teacher training program. During it, our teacher defined a Sanksrit term that made my ears perk up. *Aha*, I thought, *there is a specific word for the foolishness I have been roller-coasting through since I got back from Siberia. It's just not found in English*. It's *prajnaparada*, and it means "crimes against wisdom." And in yogic philosophy, overeating and general overindulgence constitute crimes against wisdom.

In the immense Kripalu dining hall, miniature signs have been placed at every table as reminders from the late Swami Kripalu, the founder of Kripalu yoga, to eat with *mitihar*, or moderation. "One's energy is generated, protected, and maintained by *mitihar*, which can be defined as eating the amount of food required to keep the body alert and efficient."

Was Swami Kripalu's *mitihar* an impossible ideal for ordinary humans? Upon our return to Houston, I woke up tabula rasa to make organic vegetable juice and green smoothies in the Vitamix with spirulina, papaya, kale, spinach, and almond milk. I handed D his thermoses full of Miche juice and dashed off to the Equinox gym to exercise. For lunch, I stuck to my greens. I made blended broccoli, garlic, and cilantro soup with fresh-squeezed lemon juice, practicing *mitihar* all day long. It was our dinners that were sabotaging all my efforts; nighttime was when I committed all the crimes against wisdom. By bedtime I felt as if I had treated my body like a garbage dump.

Food critics have dubbed Houston "the next culinary capital" and "the new capital of Southern cool," because of its famous foodie culture. Our house in the Montrose neighborhood sits in the epicenter of many tantalizing choices. We can walk to the institution of Italian elegance, Da Marco, or we can walk to several innovative restaurants that chef Chris Shepherd runs. Just three blocks away is Hugo's, which offers James Beard Award–winning Mexican cuisine. And I'm just getting started.

Once I returned home from Siberia, I'd recollect the months when I'd lie in bed all day and then struggle to make myself presentable to attend one of D's work dinners. To celebrate my new life—and perhaps because I'd just finished a stint of having to wear the same old yoga pants for two straight months—I now dressed up in a cocktail dress and dashed out the door to meet D. I strode through the door at Da Marco and into the old world, where waiters sporting white coats and black bowties smiled and saw me to our table.

There was a group of us gathered. The waiter brought us the chalkboard with the nightly specials written out, each one more tempting than the last. One of us fired off our customary order: a bottle of Brunello di Montalcino, roasted artichoke salad, burrata with tomatoes, and the *pièce de résistance*, risotto with white or black truffles shaved before our eyes. D would always goad the truffle-shaving waiter, "That's all we get? Put on a little more. Yeah, yeah, like that!" And the waiter would keep shaving until those revered, black-edged white truffles were heaped over our dishes of glistening risotto.

Sound decadent enough? This feast was followed by thin filets of elegant Dover sole, garnished with emerald broccoli rabe drenched in olive oil and garlic, or roasted brussels sprouts. We savored each bite. There seemed to be an unfortunate discrepancy between the delight in my mouth and the protest in my stomach.

This euphoric feeling of being lithe and light-filled in one's rejuvenated body does not last infinitely if one commits *prajnaparada* at weekly dinners. That's a humiliating understatement. As one can imagine, in spite of my earnest intentions, my body underwent vicissitudes of loss and gain. It reminded me of something I had once read: "Humans live on one-quarter of what they eat; on the other three quarters lives their doctors," which was found in an Egyptian pyramid inscription dated 3800 B.C.E.

My daytime self heeded Dr. Filonov's instructions like a renunciate, but my nocturnal self morphed into a gourmand. I had become the Jekyll and Hyde of eating. *Who was this creature?* How could I have been so careless after Dr. Filonov had worked so carefully to help me reach an optimal state of health?

Science told me that I was experiencing an opioid release of endorphins and dopamine when I overindulged, and yet even armed with this knowledge, I couldn't seem to stop these vicissitudes. And certainly, we are all faced with mine fields when it comes to eating today.

Journalist Michael Pollan has spent his career writing about the disconnection between the economic imperatives of the food industry and the biological imperatives of the human eater. As he points out, in the capitalistic food culture of America, the compulsion to overconsume is deeply psychologically entrenched, to the extent that "fully a quarter of all Americans suffer from metabolic syndrome, two thirds of us are overweight or obese, and diet-related diseases are killing the majority of us."[1]

We live in the era of ubiquitous food, which is a far cry from our ancient ancestors who had to dedicate their days to gathering enough calories to sustain life. Navigating the endless social engagements surrounding food is also a challenge for those of us trying to maintain a post-dry-fasting state of clean eating. The body has not been reprogrammed since those ancient days, though, so it protests the attempt to stay lean. I call this the primordial hormonal response to losing fat. It's a remnant from bygone days that is geared to conserve and create fat for times of need. One must be consistent in the face of biologic systems, including hormones, that are just doing their genetically programmed primordial jobs that no longer serve us, as they once did when we were in danger of starving from lack of food.

Two hormones seem particularly in play here: leptin and ghrelin. Leptin is an energy-regulating hormone that suppresses food intake and contributes to weight loss, whereas ghrelin has been dubbed the hunger hormone. Ghrelin both stimulates the appetite and signals the body to store fat. After fasting, I had a hunch that my hunger hormones were controlling me, because I had systematically eaten two to three structured meals a day without snacks for years. If only I had a laboratory to chart my dry-fasting entrances and exits; then I would have known for sure if ghrelin and leptin were the culprits.

. . .

I landed back in Siberia at the end of that summer in 2018 in hopes of seeking that ever-elusive synthesis between fasting and feasting. It was like a homecoming in Altai. The fast did not feel as peaceful as it had the first time in Siberia, though.

I wrote, "My body gets so pure, and then I pollute it as a sort of celebration. What kind of celebration is that if it taints the purity? This is not even Dionysian; it is Sader-Macher, which is the antithesis of my intention. My body is singing as loudly as a Wagnerian opera to tell me that this cannot be sustained: 'Be judicious and mindful about what you put into me. I am fond of green juices, greens, pureed soups, and salads.' I have all of the tools to be vibrant throughout my lifetime; of this I am confident." I mulled all of this over as I dry fasted and contemplated my *prajnaparada*.

As I progressed into the eighth day of my dry fast, I returned to my islet by the water for solace, and as I sat staring into my favorite stream, I thought that if my body could speak to me, it would say, "I am not a game. Be gentle and be wise with me. Don't disparage me. Treat me like something we can all be proud of: the epitome of you. Navigate wisely." I cried, thinking about how unwise I had been. *Where was wise-warrior Miche? How could I have put my newfound health in jeopardy like this?*

As I was about to exit the fast on the tenth day, I sat on the broad gray rocks by the banks of the powerful Katun river and gave it all my worries about my body and health. The vigorous turquoise rush of its waves mesmerized me, washing away my tumult. I clambered up the banks of the river back to the dirt road that I had walked countless times. My mouth was getting dry under the Siberian sun at this advanced point in my fast.

As I started up the road, I felt that familiar sense of empathy for the humans who suffer from thirst and hunger every day as the ravages of poverty, climate-change induced drought, and war-torn communities deprive them of the life-sustaining force of pure, clean water. When my family asked me for my Christmas list in 2017 after I came back from Siberia, I asked only for clean-water donations to Heifer International, a nonprofit that helps families in need throughout the world who suffer from thirst and hunger.

An epiphany came to me, and I stood still in the middle of the road. I had been feeling compassion for everyone in the world, from the chronically ill who didn't know about dry fasting to those who didn't have clean sources of water in the world and went thirsty every day. Yet I had no compassion for myself. Had I forgotten my own quirky mantra? The one I had put together in a makeshift way from my old Lyme days? "One Miche: lovable as is."

My body gave up some of its precious liquid reserves to create tears in my eyes that coursed down my dry cheeks. *Lovable as is, and that means thin or bloated, human and all.*

Had I forgotten everything? I remembered a poem attributed to Swami Kripalu (that one of his followers wrote) that is posted on the walls of Kripalu. I plunked down by the tall green thistles with raspberry centers to recite fragments of his poem aloud. It reads like this:

> My beloved child, break your heart no longer.
> Each time you judge yourself, you break your own heart;
> you stop feeding on the love which is the wellspring of your vitality.
> The time has come. Your time to live, to celebrate.
> And to see the goodness that you are.

I sat there with my eyes closed, breathing in the goodness of myself, ready to stop breaking my own heart. I wrapped my arms around myself in a makeshift hug. This exit would be a different sort of celebration, not for the healing of my physical body but for the renewed compassion for this one Miche, lovable as is.

That afternoon I received my exit orders from Sergey Ivanovich. In front of his Russian patients, he said, "Michelle is on day ten, and look how well she looks!" He said I was to break my fast alone at five a.m. by bathing in a small swimming hole set in a nook by the river. When he said that I was to exit alone, I understood how much faith and trust he had in me, for I was no longer one of his sick patients.

I squirmed all night with anticipation in my yellow sleeping bag, but at nearly four a.m. on day eleven, I couldn't wait any longer. It was August third, and I hadn't had any water since the twenty-third of July. The moon was like a lantern in the sky, and the Big Dipper was hanging right above the spot where I would be dipping my naked body. I knew that unlike those who suffer from thirst on a daily basis around the world, water was in my immediate future. I got up to prepare for this new life ahead of me; a life that included compassion for myself.

At the appointed time, I gathered all my exit paraphernalia in a basin, draped myself in my sleeping bag, slipped on my Birkenstocks, and took off purposefully down the dirt road toward the swimming hole. I spread out my sleeping bag so I could wrap up in it when I climbed out of the water. I took everything out of the basin, placed it where I thought I might need it, and put the basin just by the slim edge of the riverbank. There was nothing else to do but strip down to my naked body. I stepped into the water and thought, *It is not as cold as the Baltic*. I sat down on the rocks and started pouring water over my head. I lay back and made sure water was washing my entire body. My dehydrated body loved it, craved it. I had been staring at these rivers, dreaming of swimming in them, and here I finally was, washing off the tumult of the past months.

I knew the doctor wouldn't want me to stay in long, so I climbed out and started drying off. Then I thought, *That was just too delicious—why not do it again?* I jumped back in to swim around the tiny area and float on my back with my forehead tilted back in the rejuvenating water. I thought about the tortured months, and in a flash, I let it all go.

This all took less than a minute, but it felt like I was truly on another planet, for nothing on earth could be this exquisite. My body was happily drinking in all the water. It was pre-dawn. I was alone in a little Siberian river as if I were at one with it.

I finally climbed out to dry off and put on my exit clothes. I sat there on my sleeping bag and sipped from my thermos. I could feel all the little dry spots immediately moistening on my tongue, and the mucus breaking up. It was a defining moment in my life. I basked in compassion for the world, and for myself. I felt so free.

Later on, when the world was awake, I reflected. *Last year at the end of day nine I had ringing in my ears, weakness, and a headache. Thus far, I just feel energized.* Tania, our wonderful new cook—and, as chance would have it, my first roommate in the *dacha* two years before—brought me a cup of delicious Bolotov serum, a microflora drink that she made from Altai herbs. It was light and delicious, and full of probiotics.

I kept toasting my water to myself, lovable as is. My dear friend Natasha—who had already broken her fast—came to hug me, and Kristina came to offer her congratulations, too. D wrote, "I am very proud of your ten-day deal. Not in a way to encourage you to do aggressive things, but this is a hard thing to do." Even harder would

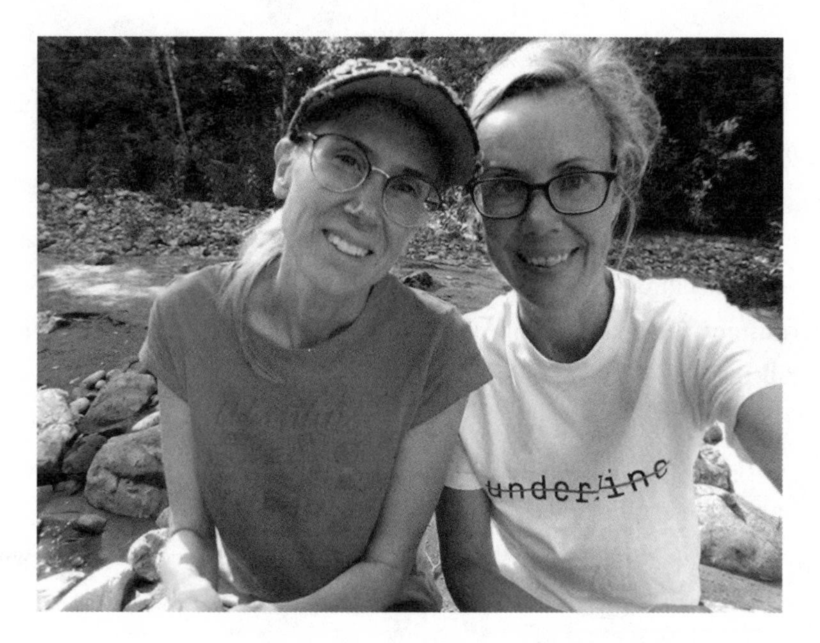

My dry-fasting sister, Natasha, and me in Siberia, summer 2018

be my intention to inflict no harm on myself. Dr. Filonov encouraged me and built me up again in Siberia; I was ready to embark on another fresh start.

. . .

My moderation while breaking that long fast brought me to form a new mantra: quality and quantity of food are equally important. In other words, it's not enough to eat organic; one must also consume modest quantities at all times. I stumbled on what Dr. Fred Bisci has to say on the subject of overeating: "By overeating, we shorten our lifespan regardless of the quality of the food. . . . Systematic undereating is the surest way of improving health."[2] A raw vegan for fifty years, Dr. Bisci had committed his own crimes against wisdom before he learned what I too had discovered with my own Sisyphean mishaps.

"When you go from having a very healthy lifestyle for a period of time and then return too quickly to an unhealthy diet, it could be more destructive than eating a consistently unhealthy diet."[3]

You can't really ever go back. That is what I've learned from my mistakes with dry fasting. You can't ever really go back to eating the way you did before—even if you thought it was healthy—and you can't ever consume the quantities of food that you once did. There is no magic pill that scientists are going to come up with to recreate autophagy. There's no shortcut to the dry-fasting methodology. For the past three years, I have maintained consistently moderate habits with food, not only while exiting but also in my quotidian nutritional routine.

My body is my temple, I kept thinking as I embarked on this new era of relationship to food. We spend so much time renovating, decorating, and cleaning our homes. You wouldn't decorate your house perfectly, wash down every surface, and then just trash it all, would you? No. Your forever home is your body. We don't have the option of leaving our bodies. Why, then, do we think we can trash our bodies to the extent that we are bloated, hungover, and miserable? I'm not scolding any readers here; I'm only sharing the run of my thoughts over my own actions.

The first yogic guideline, rendered famous by Gandhi, is the principle of *ahimsa*, or nonviolence. *Ahimsa* is not just refraining from harming others or being vegetarian; it also refers to holding back from inflicting violence on ourselves. Don't violate *ahimsa*. Take your precious body and make it like your beautiful home. Strive to cultivate at-home-ness in the body by watering it and feeding it moderately. We clear out old junk in the attic when we dry fast, and then we redecorate with healthy materials when we exit. You wouldn't renovate your house and then redecorate it with subpar junky things, would you?

In the grand microcosm of crimes against wisdom, mine were insignificant. I faithfully followed all the exit rules, and I never once overstepped the boundaries in the critical days following the dry fasts. In the enterprise of introducing safe dry fasting to you, I must share both an accidental *prajnaparada* and a common mistake I've seen beginning fasters make. After all, this chapter serves to provide a path to wisdom for you, so that you may avoid the stumbles of this dry-fasting pioneer.

Upon my return from the ten-day fast in Kaliningrad, I visited Dad and Janet in Vermont, where a *prajnaparada* was committed against me. I flew into Burlington, picked up my rental car, stopped by my favorite juice bar for supplies, and sped home. Then something started to go awry. Sitting in my jammies by Dad's bed after a flurry of hugs, I started to see horses galloping across the duvet, and it felt like puppets were holding my back up. I crawled to the living room sofa where there was an imaginary child leading me down a hole into a story, and then into another scene. I was laughing and crying and rocking, and suddenly I was in the kitchen tearing open a box of gluten-free crackers.

I knew that I was out of control, but I didn't know how to stop it. To my alarmed parents, I said, "Something is happening, and I can see it, but I have no control!"

"Michael, I think that this is what they call sky high," I could hear Janet nervously reporting to Dad.

Dad called the juice bar, and I could hear him frantically asking, "What did you give my daughter?" He discovered that the large lemon, coconut oil, honey, and hot water herbal concoction I had sipped all the way home was full of CBD oil. It wasn't marked, and I would never have consumed oil of marijuana of my own accord, and here I had just come out of a ten-day dry fast. My body was as pure as it gets.

I could hear Dad saying loudly, "My daughter is tripping on Happy Tea?" It was funny and not funny, and I couldn't do anything about it. Janet was fluttering around me, never having seen anyone high before. She helped me get to bed, and I slept it off over sixteen uninterrupted hours. When I woke up, I was in a state of bliss until I remembered.

I padded out right away to let them know I was okay. As Janet put it, "This was not the reunion we had all been anticipating." The owner of the juice bar told Dad that CBD oil doesn't get anyone high because it doesn't have THC in it, but that I had the last cup of it, so the dredges had the most concentrated amount of CBD. Dad explained to her that I had come off a dry fast. When I told Dr. Filonov that morning, he was exasperated: "Your body is so pure—you must be very careful!" Although I didn't mean to make this frightful faux pas, I recommend that you avoid such substances at all costs, particularly straight after a long dry fast.

The other avoidable misstep that I've seen many people new to fasting make is filling up on heavy food directly before and after the fast. It's a natural impulse, but tapering slowly in and out of the fast on only fruit and vegetables is critical. I have read books in which even doctors, writing about their own experiments with short-term fasts, recount gorging on steak the night before a fast, and then breaking it with bacon and eggs. Please don't ever follow in their misguided footsteps, for this is a violent affront to the body that is attempting to clean itself out.

Some patients have fretfully asked me if they will ruin their fasts by overeating afterward. They worry that they will fall back into the abyss of Lyme. Fret not, you may feel like a bloated mess if you overeat one day, but you can always water fast or dry fast for one or two days if you overindulge.

You will never fall back into Lyme. Dry fasts are cumulative, so you cannot ever go back to your original starting point. This is a radically different treatment than any of the ones that you have undergone before, and flare-ups are not part of the post-dry-fasting life, even if human ups and downs definitely are—particularly when primal hunger strikes.

After a few long rounds of dry fasting and exiting, I no longer have waves of cravings fueled by pesky hunger hormones. Cravings are ephemeral, and they will pass. I learned to master cravings by turning to my meditative breathing techniques. My Kripalu teachers like Rudy Pierce teach an invaluable tool called BRFWA (pronounced "burfwa"), which stands for breathe, relax, feel, watch, allow. Through breathing calmly, relaxing in the midst of an inner emotional storm, and watching it as a detached observer without reacting to it, I cultivate an inner witness that allows me to tolerate distressing emotions without turning to a destructive habit like emotional eating.

However, on the wise warrior's path, at dusk, when the light is dim, I may trip on a pebble that looks an awful lot like wild mushroom risotto, or it may sprinkle a vintage Barolo one evening. When that happens, I brush myself off with compassion and get right back on the path. As Kripalu's unofficial poet laureate Danna Faulds writes in this excerpt from her poem "Allow":

> There is no controlling life.
> Try corralling a lightning bolt,
> containing a tornado. Dam a
> stream and it will create a new
> channel. Resist, and the tide
> will sweep you off your feet.

> Allow, and grace will carry
> you to higher ground. The only
> safety lies in letting it all in—
> the wild with the weak; fear,
> fantasies, failures and success. . . .[4]

Although I embrace the vicissitudes of life, I'm confident that my pendulum swings happen within the healthy parameters I learned from Dr. Filonov. I am at peace knowing that I can stay on my healthy path for life while having the grace to still live with freedom and spontaneity.

EPILOGUE

I nearly needed to die to live again. Long after my healing, Kristina told Dr. Filonov that I had planned to commit assisted suicide if dry fasting didn't eradicate my disease. Kristina urged me to show him two photos that I had spliced side by side. The one on the left shows me languishing, before I came to Siberia for the first time, and the second shows me whirling out of Altai two months later like a swell in the Katun river. Dr. Filonov exclaimed, "The light had gone out of your eyes. But look at your light now." He knows he saved my life.

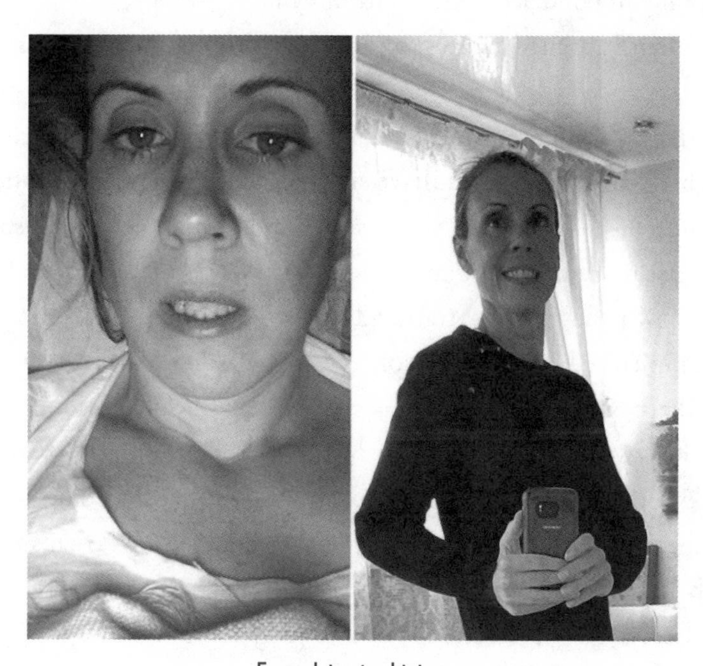

From dying to shining

One year after my first return from Siberia, I celebrated my new birthday in life by hiking the Vermont portion of the Appalachian Trail in less than a week. D dropped me off at the Appalachian Trail head in North Adams, Massachusetts. Over the next several days, I hiked an average of thirty miles a day from dawn to dark, proclaiming to myself, *I'm definitely not a sick girl! No, not me! Not with this mileage. I'm Lyme-free Miche!*

Hiking in humid 85-degree weather with a ten-kilo backpack made me think I needed to revisit the definition of celebration. I had spent so many years in Lyme disease mud that it did not exactly feel like a celebration when my blue hiking shoes turned brown with mud, or when mud splattered all the way up my thighs. In my quest to travel ultralight, I didn't pack a camp shirt, so I hiked fifteen hours a day in a sweaty long-sleeved base layer that I peeled off at night in my tent. There were a few transcendent moments, nonetheless, and I had time to ponder my lessons from Lyme.

When I reached the top of Stratton Mountain, I was drenched in sweat and my long tick-proof hiking pants clung to my wet legs. A Green Mountain Club caretaker named Jean—she should be dubbed Saint Jean—must have smelled me coming, for she offered me one of her orange GMC T-shirts and two apples her husband had just picked. It was a meaningful birthday gift, and I ran all the way down the trail to Stratton Pond for a sunset skinny dip. The pond mirrored the sky's salmon and periwinkle hues as I swam.

The next morning, as I was standing on Bromley Mountain at sunrise, sweatily basking in the mist over the forest-green Vermont peaks, I thought about the ways in which Lyme had ended up being a gift because it taught me so many lessons. I had always been smitten with Swami Kripalu's statement that "the highest form of spiritual practice is self-observation without judgment," but I spent years failing to live by those words. Lyme accomplished this for me even as it flattened me.

Lyme forced me to release my perfectionistic proclivities, creating the condition in which, immobilized and broken, I had to accept my "One Miche, lovable as is" mantra. I was not completely unproductive because I was doing deep inner work. For the first time in my life, I observed my state without judging it. Perhaps my immune system had become susceptible because I drove myself so hard all the time to succeed in my academic career, to the extent that I lost that same career. Letting go of being a perfectionist, post-Lyme, I gained serenity for the first time. Now I could appreciate the sunrise on top of Bromley without racing on to the next leg. I had learned to build reserves of energy and channel energy wisely, rather than sap it quickly. I had learned to stop being so anxious about failing when I embarked on a big project. Dry fasting also had shown me how strong and hardy I really am, and it gave me the gift of self-confidence that I had never possessed before. As I hiked on toward Killington, I repeated, *I am resilient. I am whole. I am worthy. I am healthy*. And what's more, I believed all those words.

When I emerged from the woods, 125 miles later, D was just about to pull off the highway, so I hitchhiked to the Inn at Long Trail for lunch. When D came up to the hiker's bar and saw my mud-spattered legs and sweaty face he cracked, "Look at the RGO!" We roared with laughter and high-fived to protect his dress shirt. We kept on driving to celebrate my new birthday with Dad and Janet, farther up the Vermont corridor. Janet opened the door said, "We are so proud of our little faster turned hiker!" I flew into Dad's arms, and he whispered, "My precious Michelley is back in business!" Later, Dad offered an alluring thought for the future, "One of these days you will surely make it to the top of your Mt. Belukha in Siberia.

That's *possible* now." Dad marveled at the return of his mountain goat. Starving in Siberia had enabled me to live again like the carpe diem girl I once was. Dad, D, and Janet got their girl back.

It had happened because I decided to be healthy. One cannot ever be truly well if one continues to identify as a sick person. In my new life, I never tell people I meet that I was ever ill, unless I need to explain the gaps in my adult life, those periods for which I have nothing on my CV.

I've written this book because I know I'm not an anomaly. We all have the innate capacity for cellular rejuvenation. But so far, it's largely untapped. Shed the toxic label "sick." While I was dry fasting in Siberia the first time, I fell on this formidable Rumi poem that imperatively told me to "take an axe to the prison wall. Escape. Walk out like someone suddenly born into color. Do it now."[1] I did it, and now I am giving you the most powerful axe that you will ever receive to break out of the Lyme prison for good.

The Lyme patients I have met and coached all led extraordinary lives before the disease extinguished their light. Each one was in possession of a vitality that, while it had grown dulled by illness, shone once again after dry fasting.

Your body carries inherent knowledge in the DNA of your cells—the fountain of youth has rested heretofore latent within your own body. You are a pioneer when you start dry fasting. If you embark on this journey, you will discover a resilience within that will make you soar. As the ageless wisdom of the *Upanishads* imparts, "Joy comes from being in harmony with the creative forces of the universe," and it can be so for all of us if we cleanse our body, mind, and spirit in quest of an extraordinary new normal.[2] Today, my joy comes from spending quality screen-free time with animals, friends, and family, hiking in the mountains, running nimbly to happy songs, playing my musical instruments, and writing books that could make a meaningful impact on others' lives. It means being less connected to the internet so that I can *be* and *savor* the beauty in this world. My journey—as epic for me as the adventures of J.R.R. Tolkien's hobbits were for them—has brought me back to my Micheness, my joy, and my vitality. I share it so that you, too, may find your ipseity—that which makes your spark within *inherently you.*

I wanted to write a memoir on recovering from a debilitating illness that robbed me of my cognitive faculties, my creativity, and my ability to function in what became a decrepit physical body. I felt compelled to write this memoir and handbook for dry fasting because thousands—if not millions—of people could be helped by my experiences. I felt a moral obligation to write it and share it widely to pay it forward. Once you are rejuvenated by the scientific miracle of autophagy that Dr. Filonov has perfected, please pay it forward, too. *Na Zdarovie*—to your health.

APPENDIX A: MEDITATIONS FOR DRY FASTING

For the thirty days before you begin fasting, start keeping a journal. Record your hopes, fears, and feelings surrounding healing. While you're fasting, record the epiphanies that come to you.

Preparatory Meditation: Taking Stock

Find a quiet place to sit comfortably with an erect spine, with your sitz bones on the floor and your hips raised above your knees. If you need to sit on a cushion, please do so. You may also sit on a chair with an erect spine. Close your eyes and start to take slow breaths through your nose. For four long counts, inhale and direct the breath toward your belly, your rib cage, and your upper chest. Pause. Exhale for four slow, long counts.

As you begin to make this breathing exercise a steady, rhythmical pattern, start to notice if there are any body parts that are holding tension, including your muscles, chest, jaw, shoulders, and so forth. Each time that you exhale, imagine softening these areas and releasing the tension. You may even say silently to yourself, "With each exhalation, I release anything that is not serving me right now."

Each time that you inhale, imagine inhaling a sense of peace that brings you to stillness and quiet. This sense of peace is individualized and may be whatever you find spiritual—it may be derived from religion, nature, music, poetry, the energy of the universe, or whatever resonates with you as a deep place of safety, comfort, and quiet. Each time that a thought enters your mind, acknowledge it, and let it go. Direct your mind back toward the simple process of inhaling slowly and exhaling slowly. Do not judge yourself for having a thought; merely observe the thought, let it go, and keep returning your attention to the breath. If it helps, imagine your favorite river or stream, and imagine putting that thought into the river and watching it float away. With each inhalation, imagine breathing in healing energy, and with each exhalation, watch the tensions in your body melt and soften. Once you have come to a quiet place, begin to direct your attention to taking stock of your life.

By taking stock of your life, I mean: Where are you right now? Where would you like to be? What is serving you well about your life? What is not serving you well that you would like to shift, alter, eliminate, or change? As you breathe, with your eyes closed, relying on the pattern of the breath to soothe you, go deep within and examine what is true for you right now. Watch, listen, and observe as if you are a witness of your own life, without judgment, without frustration. Merely watch and observe what comes up for you. It may be something that seems blatantly obvious, such as "I am chronically ill and no longer want to be." It may be "I no longer want to feel inadequate and insecure." "I no longer want to be in a toxic relationship with Person A." "I love teaching and want to organize my life so that I can do more of it." Whatever comes up for you, simply observe it. If something painful comes up, acknowledge the distress, try to listen to any message it is giving you, and inhale compassion for this pain. Exhale and breathe out the pain without judging it.

After a while, you may want to open your eyes and start writing down anything important that has come to you during this process. You may want to repeat this process every day during the preparatory period of fasting.

Vision Board

"What is my dream for my post-fasting life—my new normal?" Use a large piece of paper or a section of your journal to create a vision board for yourself. What are the parts of your life that you love and would like to cultivate more? What are the parts of your life that are not serving you well and you would like to let go of? If you were not ill, what would you like to do? Who would you like to be? Use your imagination and dream about your new normal as a well person. You may continue working on this during the fasting period, and during each exit period. Dream what may have once been an "impossible dream." It may be as simple as writing out: "Cello," "Nature," "Dogs," "Volunteering," or "Yoga."

"Letting Go" Meditation

Repeat the first breathing exercise above. Then focus on "letting go of my identity as a sick person." If the prospect of this is frightening, you might go deep within and ask yourself why you are holding on to this piece of your identity? See what you can let go of as you allow yourself to stay in the safe place of examining your thoughts and feelings. Whatever you can let go of, cast it into a river that carries it away from you. Imagine filling yourself up with healing light that shines on all the dark places that need healing.

Sankalpa Meditation: Setting an Intention

Set your thought and energy on a pure hope for your dry fast to heal you. Close your eyes, inhale slowly through your nose (or mouth if necessary), and exhale through your mouth. As you breathe, shed any pressure or fear you may be feeling before you fast. As you come to a place of stillness, formulate a positive intention for your fast and hold steadfast to the thought throughout the fasting period, repeating it as you walk and as you breathe.

Pulse Meditation: "I Cast My Burden"

One meditation that I find helpful while dry fasting, if I'm experiencing aches and pains or emotional sensitivity, is a pulse meditation. I sit in a comfortable seated position with my eyes closed and take my pulse with one wrist pressing into the other. I identify my "burden"—that is, whatever stress or anxiety is weighing on my mind. On each beat of my heart, I say in time, "I cast my burden on *my higher self*, and I go free." Alternatively, replace "my higher self" with "God," or "on the river," or whatever you wish. I find this to be tremendously powerful and calming.

"I Am" Meditation

Coming to a quiet, still place and using your breath to guide you, pause and imagine what you would most like to manifest for yourself. Devise a succinct "I am" mantra for yourself. It may be as simple as "I am healthy, I am." "I am shining and bouncing, I am." "I am a successfully published author, I am." "I am well, I am." "I am a positive person, I am." Whatever it may be, practice it throughout your fasting practice morning and night.

APPENDIX B:
FASTING PROTOCOL

Performing the Fasts

Twenty-four-hour water fast: If you are water fasting, only consume water starting at bedtime on the day before your fast and continue to consume only water until the morning after your fast. For instance, water fast from a Thursday night to a Saturday morning.

If your twenty-four-hour water fast takes place easily, allow yourself to recover for one week, and repeat the water fast for *three days*. Exit the water fast for one week, and engage in a *seven-day* water fast. After a successful seven-day water fast, you may begin a twenty-four-hour dry fast.

Twenty-four-hour dry fast: Consume water only on the day preceding your fast. Your fast will begin at bedtime. For instance, if fasting on a Saturday, the dry fast will begin Friday night at bedtime, and you will continue dry fasting until you wake up on Sunday morning.

Three-day dry fast: Use the same principle of the twenty-four-hour dry fast to proceed with the three-day fast. Your fast will begin at bedtime, for example, on a Thursday, and you will not consume any food or water from Thursday night until Monday morning. During this time, do not apply any lotions, do not brush your teeth or wash your face, and do not come in contact with any water. If you experience headaches, dry mouth, nausea, hunger, or thirst, breathe through them, for they will pass and shift. A multitude of symptoms is normal while dry fasting. The better your preparation is, the easier you will fast.

Five-, six-, seven-, eight-, nine-day dry fast: Incrementally add days to your dry-fasting protocol. Many people jump from three days to nine days while dry fasting in Siberia, but I recommend advancing from three days to five days. On the fractional program that Dr. Filonov recommends, the resting period should be at least the equivalent of the fasting period. Hence, a three-day fast should be followed by a minimum three-day exit. No one should conduct a fast for nine days without consulting with Dr. Filonov.

• • •

While fasting, try to walk as much as possible during the day. Spend time outdoors in nature and avoid dry places such as those heated with electric heaters. Allow yourself to rest fully; do not plan to work, to drive, or to engage in any activities that involve lifting weight, excessive talking, or intellectually stimulating reading. Try to engage in a digital detox from your phone and computer so that your mind can rest.

While fasting, incorporate the breathing technique described above. Spend at least ten minutes every morning and every evening engaging in long, slow, deep inhalations and exhalations in a quiet space with your eyes closed. Imagine inhaling cleansing, healing light into every part of your body, methodically, slowly. Exhale the tension, pain, and anxiety from your body and mind, slowly and methodically. Release your thoughts and invite your mind to rest during this critical healing period. Let yourself reside in the quiet, suspended space of peace for as long as you can.

While fasting, enumerate the things in your life for which you are grateful. Generate this positive energy whether it is for the fasting process, your family, the lessons you learned from the illness, the trees, the flowers, the animals, and so on.

Exiting the Fasts

Twenty-four-hour/three-day/seven-day water fast: You may consume a small piece of fruit (other than citrus) in the morning, therapeutically chewing each bite thirty times, or until it's pulverized into juice. For lunch, you may consume one cup of finely chopped broom salad, which is named for the intestinal sweep that it initiates. Broom salad may include broccoli, fennel, red cabbage, carrot, celery, or any mixture of fibrous, cruciferous vegetables that you have on hand. Juice one half of a lemon into your salad, but avoid oil and salt for at least three days. For dinner, you may repeat the broom salad or have one cup of steamed vegetables or vegetable soup. On the second day, you may incorporate a small portion of fish such as salmon or cod, avoiding high-mercury fish like tuna and swordfish, etc. Gradually experiment with introducing foods back into your diet. You may also have a small portion of cooked millet for breakfast, or buckwheat kasha. Or you may prefer to maintain an exclusively raw-food diet while you are on the fasting protocol. Listen to your individual body's needs rather than following a structured protocol that someone else has devised.

Twenty-four-hour dry fast: In the morning, take a cold shower to break your dry fast. Prepare a thermos of hot water (tea temperature) and slowly sip the hot water until noon. Only have hot water—no cold water—for two days. Prepare a small pot of compote and slowly sip it until evening (see Appendix C for recipes). In the evening, you may have a piece of watermelon or apple—no citrus the first day—and therapeutically chew each bite until it is pulverized into a juice before you swallow it. On the second day, you may use the protocol for breaking the water fast. If you experience any nausea or headache, take two activated charcoal tablets on an empty stomach, and drink one teaspoon of baking soda in hot water.

Three-day dry fast: Break the fast as you would for the twenty-four-hour dry fast; however, you may listen to your body's hunger cues to see if you are ready for fruit on the first day or if you need a twenty-four-hour period of hot water.

Seven-day/nine-day dry fast: Do not brush your teeth with toothpaste or use any lotions or soaps for the first twenty-four hours; break the fast in an ice-cold bath by dumping a basin of cold water over your head. Prepare a thermos of hot water, and slowly sip from it for twenty-four hours. Do not consume anything else. After twenty-four hours, continue with the hot water, as much as your body needs, and assess whether you need an additional twenty-four hours or more of hot water, or whether you are ready to incorporate compote and vegetable broth. Then continue gradually introducing the fruit, broom salad, steamed vegetables, kasha, and fish in small portions.

Make sure to take at least seven days to exit in this manner for a seven-day dry fast, and twenty-one days for a nine-day dry fast.

Consume small portions of high-quality, nutrient-dense meals. Avoid oil, salt, and excess fats. Do not consume any meat for one month. Allow your body to rest deeply during the exit and continue your breathing exercises. Continue to walk as much as you can; allow yourself to sleep deeply; do not judge any physical or mental fatigue during the critical exit period. Allow yourself at least three weeks of rest and healing.

APPENDIX C: MICHELLE'S SUNLIGHT FOODS RECIPES

Eating nourishing, organic meals is practicing good self-care. Your food is your medicine, providing the optimum fuel for your body. I encourage you to revise and improvise the recipes here as you wish.

Recommended Kitchen Tools:

- Vitamix blender: You can sometimes find these sold used or refurbished.
- Juicer: I use a simple Breville fountain juicer.
- Hand-held vegetable chopper: I like the Chef'n VeggiChop Hand-Powered Food Chopper, but it has a limited capacity to make portions for more than one person.
- Large soup pot
- Small bowl: I like to choose a pretty ceramic or wooden bowl to eat my meals in, in a size that helps with portion control.
- Good paring knife: I use a simple Waring knife.
- Nut milk bag: This is optional but useful for those who want to make homemade almond milk, etc.

Sample Grocery List:

Note: All produce should be organic.

Apples
Blueberries
Watermelon
Lemons
Grapefruits
Turmeric root (fresh)
Ginger root (fresh)
Garlic
Red onions
Beets
Kale
Spinach
Parsley
Dill
Cucumbers
Tomatoes
Red cabbage
Fennel
Broccoli
Zucchini
Green beans
Cauliflower
Romaine lettuce
Coconut oil
Olive oil
Tahini
Artichoke hearts
Arugula
Coconut water (preferably a raw organic refrigerated variety)

Peas (frozen peas are okay)
Wild-caught salmon
Wild-caught cod
Millet
Buckwheat kasha (green, not roasted)
Cardamom
Cinnamon
Almonds (raw, if possible)
Herbal tea (chamomile, peppermint, etc.)
Spirulina powder, chlorella powder, and raw cacao powder (optional)
Bananas
Alternative milk (oat, buckwheat, hemp, almond, rice, etc.)
Flaxseed oil
Hemp seeds
Frozen raw coconut meat (available from Exotic Superfoods)
Brad's cheddar raw veggie chips (available from Whole Foods or internet)

Very Special Indispensable Ingredients:

- Gratitude for the nourishing food and liquids
- A generous measure of self-love

Miche's Green Juices

Juice any combination of the following ingredients, using cucumber, celery, or romaine lettuce as a base. Plan to juice sixteen ounces.

Celery, cucumber, ginger, lemon
Carrot, celery, apple, lemon, ginger

Romaine, celery, lemon, ginger, parsley
Romaine, kale, parsley, fennel, lemon
Celery, tomato, lemon
Beet, ginger, lemon, apple, parsley (add one teaspoon of flax oil and shake)

Be creative; invent your own combination of nearly any veggies. Note that kale doesn't yield much juice and that broccoli is an intense juicing experience—not 101. Try to limit fruits in the juices, as Dr. Filonov argues that the fruit should largely be eaten, not juiced, to avoid overloading the pancreas. If you like, you can strain your juice into a glass Ball jar and consume within a few minutes. Fresh juice does not keep long.

Miche's Healing Homemade Veggie Broth

Wash and cut up one potato, one onion, two carrots, two stalks of celery, and one beet, and add chopped parsley. Fill your pot with spring water (non-chlorinated), and bring it to a boil for ten minutes. Reduce the heat so that it simmers for thirty minutes. Consume only the broth—no solids. This is a nourishing experience for the body after dry fasting.

Spring Green Veggie Broth

Wash and cut up three cups of kale, three cups of spinach, one cup of peas (fresh or frozen) three tablespoons of fresh turmeric root, three tablespoons of fresh ginger root, three tablespoons of parsley, and two tablespoons of coconut oil. Add all ingredients to a large soup pot as you chop them. Fill the soup pot with at least two to three quarts of fresh spring water.

Keep the heat on a low setting so that the mixture simmers for thirty to sixty minutes, depending on your time constraints in the kitchen. Do not bring to a boil. With a ladle, put three cups of the mixture into your Vitamix blender, and blend until everything is smoothly combined. Your broth will have a spring green color. You may consume the broth for breakfast, lunch, or dinner, and you may also consume the vegetables in the broth. Do not add any additional seasonings or oil.

Miche's Swamp Juice

In your Vitamix, put one teaspoon or more of spirulina powder, chlorella powder, and raw cacao powder. Add one frozen banana. (I like to buy a bunch or two of ripe bananas, peel them, break them into pieces, and put them in a glass storage container to freeze them for smoothies.)

Add one cup of spinach or arugula, or even cilantro, which is one of our household favorites.

Add at least one cup of nut milk or more if desired—enough to create your desired consistency. Blend at high speed until the mixture is smooth; consume it immediately.

Homemade Almond Milk

Soak one to two pounds of organic raw almonds overnight in a bowl full of spring water. In the morning, drain the water and rinse the almonds. Place them in the Vitamix blender with two cups of spring water per pound of almonds. You may add one to two dates to the mixture, taking care to de-pit them. Blend the mixture on high speed until it's smooth. (I blend them for at least two minutes.) Place your nut milk bag over a wide-mouth container. Gradually pour the blended almond mixture from the Vitamix into the nut milk bag. Squeeze the bag so that the almond milk comes out cleanly into the wide-mouth container. I like to use glass Ball jars. Add desired spices, such as cardamom, vanilla, cinnamon, or nutmeg. Drop in a few grains of Himalayan sea salt if desired. Cover the wide-mouth container with a lid and shake the almond milk with the added spices. Consume within a few days.

Dr. Filonov's Russian Compote "Exit Juice"

The cooks at Dr. Filonov's center in Altai don't use measuring cups. The best way to make compote is to size up your pot. I encourage you to use a small pot the first time, and add two chopped apples, or two chopped pears, and either a few dried apricots or a handful of blueberries and raisins. These fruits work best. Then fill up your pot with spring water. If you have two cups of cut fruit, perhaps aim to add four cups of water. Cover the mixture, bring it to a boil, and then turn the temperature down to let it simmer for thirty minutes or longer. You can even let it simmer on very low heat for a couple of hours, as they do in Siberia. Only consume the compote juice, and make sure that it's served hot. This nutritious liquid is essential for rebuilding glycogen stores during exits from extended fasts. I find that a little goes a long way, but the Russian patients say, "The more *Kompot*, the better!"

Miche's Chopped Broom Salad

In your hand-held vegetable chopper, add the following: one half cup of coarsely chopped red cabbage, one half cup of coarsely chopped fennel, one half cup of coarsely chopped greens (such as kale, spinach, cilantro, arugula, etc.), one medium beet, three tablespoons of parsley, and one half of a peeled and deseeded lemon. Optionally, you can add one half of an avocado. Tightly close the cap on the vegetable chopper, and pull the cord at least twenty times to chop the vegetables until they are very finely grated. Enjoy plain if you're on the first days of your exit from fasting. Take care to therapeutically chew even though the salad is finely chopped. If you have passed the critical early exit period, then you may add a few grains of Himalayan pink sea salt, a tablespoon of extra virgin olive oil, or a tablespoon of tahini to the chopper before you begin pulling the string. That way, they will be nicely blended into your broom salad. Enjoy as often as you wish!

Variations: Include any vegetables from the sample grocery list to this mixture that you may be craving. The body may have a certain request that you may wish to honor.

Garnish: You may wish to chop half of an avocado to place on top of your salad before you consume it.

Miche's Million-Dollar Sunlight Foods Salad

During my lengthy raw vegan period, I invited my cousins for dinner one night. They were used to dining in Michelin-starred establishments throughout the globe, and they said, "Michelle, you could make a million dollars with this salad!" This salad is the staple of my diet, along with my broom salad, and it changes according to the seasonal organic vegetables I find at my local farmers' markets.

Chop:

3 tbsp. raw cabbage
1 head of fennel
1 cup of sprouts (broccoli sprouts are my favorite, but alfalfa or any other sprouts will work)
½ cup dandelion greens (if available in the spring)
1 endive
1 cup lacinato kale

1–3 tbsp. of fresh herbs (preferably cilantro, since it has potent chelation properties and helps expel heavy metals from the body)

You may have to make this in batches in the chopper and then toss the ingredients chopped into a large salad bowl. Mix all the ingredients together in the salad bowl, then add the following ingredients, which should be hand-cut, not chopped in the vegetable chopper:

1 avocado chopped in cubes
2 tbsp. sundried tomatoes
½ cup (or more if you like) of artichoke hearts (I prefer the marinated buffalo artichokes from Whole Foods)
2 tbsp. Kalamata olives (raw if possible)
3 tbsp. raw, organic, non-GMO hemp seeds

Toss with Miche's Salad Dressing, and top with Brad's cheddar raw veggie chips.

Miche's Salad Dressing

Mix the following (which makes one serving; adjust quantities for more) with a whisk:

2 tbsp. raw, organic tahini
3 tbsp. extra virgin olive oil
Juice of 1 lemon
Dash of Himalayan sea salt
Touch of cayenne pepper or turmeric powder (if desired)

Blend to your desired consistency, and toss with Miche's salad.

Raw Carrot Avocado Ginger Soup

Chop one cup of carrots, and blend in the Vitamix with one avocado, one clove of garlic, one tablespoon of ginger juice (juiced in juicer), one tablespoon of lemon juice, and a dash of Himalayan pink sea salt. If you are at least five days out of your dry fast, you may add a touch of cayenne pepper or a touch of cumin and coriander powder to make it curried soup. Blend with at least one cup of hot water, or add more if you like a watery soup. This nutritious soup serves one person.

Fennel Gazpacho

In the Vitamix, blend one entire bulb of fennel with one clove of garlic, one avocado, and half of a cucumber. You might also add one half cup of cherry tomatoes if lectins and nightshade vegetables and fruits do not aggravate your digestive system. Add one cup of water and lemon juice, if desired. Blend until smooth, and garnish with fresh herbs—cilantro or parsley would be nice choices.

Miche's Garlic Broccoli Soup

This is a warm, cooked, nourishing soup for the winter or for a heartier meal.

Steam two cups of broccoli for five minutes until it is cooked al dente. Pour both the broccoli and the water in which it was steamed into the Vitamix. Add one cup of cilantro, one to three cloves of garlic, the juice of one lemon, and a dash of sea salt. Blend until smooth (at least two minutes). Enjoy warm!

Dr. Filonov's Fish Soup

Dr. Filonov finds fish soup to be a nourishing, healing meal to be enjoyed during the up-building phase of the exit. His wife, Valentina, and his cook Tania make exceptional versions of this soup. Wash and chop two carrots, two stalks of celery, one potato, one leek, and one cup of dill. Add these to a medium-sized soup pot with one tablespoon of extra virgin olive oil, two bay leaves, and a dash of Himalayan sea salt. Turn the heat to medium for three to five minutes, and stir the ingredients with a wooden spoon until the olive oil is coating the vegetables and they are starting to soften. Add one quart of spring water and one to two pounds of cod with the skin removed. It will break apart into pieces. Bring the soup to a boil for one minute, and then turn the heat to medium low so that the soup can simmer until the vegetables are soft and the fish is cooked. Do not overcook; the vegetables and fish should preserve their vitality. Enjoy this nourishing soup from Siberia.

Frozen Coconut Cream with Cardamom

Even Dad, the Ben & Jerry's aficionado, lights up with delight when I take a package of frozen coconut meat out of the freezer. This is a win that is sugar-free and has antimicrobial properties in the coconut.

Allow one package of frozen meat from Exotic Superfoods to semi-thaw until there are still some frozen chunks but it is pliable. Add it to the Vitamix along with one half to one cup of either coconut water or coconut milk. Season with your favorite spices. Mine are one teaspoon of cardamom, one teaspoon of vanilla, and one pitted date (optional). Cinnamon and nutmeg are also delicious choices. If you are feeling decadent, you may even add two tablespoons of raw cacao to your treat (not to be confused or substituted with cocoa powder). Blend the ingredients in the Vitamix until you achieve your desired consistency. Place the mixture in serving-size containers, and freeze it partially. If you allow it to freeze entirely, it will be quite solid and take some time to thaw.

Night Caps and Morning Potions

Better Beet It: For a nice warm morning drink, juice one beet, one to two inches of ginger root, and one lemon. Add one cup of hot water, and mix it all together with a spoon.

Chamomile Thyme: Boil a quart of water, and pour it over a fresh bunch of thyme leaves and two tablespoons of dried loose-leaf chamomile. Let it steep for ten minutes. Strain it through a sieve into your cup with a squeeze of lemon or with local, organic honey. It's always chamomile time for me.

NOTES

Introduction

1. However, ticks have existed for millions of years and have a long history of infecting humans and animals.
2. Centers for Disease Control and Prevention, "Lyme Disease," October 1, 2020, https://www.cdc.gov/ticks/tickbornediseases/lyme.html.
3. John J. Halperin, "Neurologic Manifestations of Lyme Disease," *Current Infectious Disease Reports* 13, no. 4 (2011): 360–366.
4. American Autoimmune Related Diseases Association, "Autoimmune Facts," accessed February 15, 2022, https://autoimmune.org/wp-content/uploads/2019/12/1-in-5-Brochure.pdf.
5. National Institutes of Health, "Progress in Autoimmune Diseases Research," March 2005, https://www.niaid.nih.gov/sites/default/files/adccfinal.pdf.
6. Lihua Duan, Xiaoquan Rao, and Keshav Raj Sigdel, "Regulation of Inflammation in Autoimmune Disease," *Journal of Immunology Research*, February 28, 2019, https://doi.org/10.1155/2019/7403796.
7. Mathilde Versini, Pierre-Yves Jeandel, Eric Rosenthal, and Yehuda Shoenfeld, "Obesity in Autoimmune Diseases: Not a Passive Bystander," *Autoimmunity Reviews* 13, no. 9 (2014): 981–1000.
8. Sergey Filonov, *Dry Fasting: 20 Questions and Answers* (Moscow: Siberika, 2019), 56.

Chapter 1

1. Amy Tan, *The Opposite of Fate: A Book of Musings* (New York: G. P. Putnam's Sons, 2003), 367.
2. Joseph Romm, *Climate Change: What Everyone Needs to Know* (Oxford: Oxford University Press, 2015), 1.

3. Alison F. Hinckley, Neeta P. Connally, James I. Meek, Barbara J. Johnson, Melissa M. Kemperman, Katherine A. Feldman, Jennifer L. White, and Paul S. Mead, "Lyme Disease Testing by Large Commercial Laboratories in the United States," *Clinical Infectious Diseases* 59, no. 5 (2014): 676–681.

4. Steven Phillips and Dana Parish, *Chronic: The Hidden Cause of the Autoimmune Pandemic and How to Get Healthy Again* (New York: Houghton Mifflin Harcourt, 2020), 204.

Chapter 2

1. Meghan O'Rourke, *Sun in Days: Poems* (New York: W. W. Norton, 2017), 119.

2. Louise Bazalgette, William Bradley, and Jenny Ousbey, *The Truth about Suicide* (London: Demos, 2011).

Chapter 4

1. Virginia Woolf, *On Being Ill* (Ashfield, MA: Paris Press, 2012), 7; Ludwig Wittgenstein, *Philosophical Investigations*, trans. G. E. M. Anscombe (Oxford: Blackwell, 2001), §253.

Chapter 7

1. Rumi, "By the Sound of Their Voice," in *The Rumi Collection*, ed. Kabir Helminski (London: Shambhala, 2012), 4.

Chapter 8

1. Rachel Carson, *Silent Spring* (New York: Houghton Mifflin, 2002), 8.

2. Wendell Berry, *New Collected Poems* (Berkeley, CA: Counterpoint Press, 2012).

3. Rumi, *The Analects of Rumi*, ed. Akṣapāda (n.p.: independently published, 2019), 123.

Chapter 14

1. E. E. Cummings, "i thank You God for most this amazing," in *Complete Poems, 1904–1962*, ed. George James Firmage (New York: Liveright, 2008).

Chapter 16

1. Centers for Disease Control and Prevention, "How Many People Get Lyme Disease?" January 13, 2021, https://www.cdc.gov/lyme/stats/humancases.html.
2. Johns Hopkins Bloomberg School of Public Health, "Lyme Disease Costs Up to $1.3 Billion per Year, Study Finds," February 5, 2015, https://publichealth.jhu.edu/2015/lyme-disease-costs-more-than-one-billion-dollars-per-year-to-treat-study-finds.
3. Johns Hopkins Bloomberg School of Public Health, "Lyme Disease Costs."
4. Robert C. Bransfield, "Suicide and Lyme and Associated Diseases," *Neuropsychotic Disease and Treatment* 13 (2017): 1575–1587.
5. Gina Kolata and Sewell Chan, "Yoshinori Ohsumi of Japan Wins Nobel Prize for Study of 'Self-Eating' Cells," *New York Times*, October 3, 2016, https://www.nytimes.com/2016/10/04/science/yoshinori-ohsumi-nobel-prize-medicine.html.
6. Mark Mattson, "Why Fasting Bolsters Brain Power," TEDx Talks, March 18, 2014, https://www.youtube.com/watch?v=4UkZAwKoCP8.
7. Anahad O'Connor, "Fasting Diets Are Gaining Acceptance," *New York Times*, March 7, 2016, https://well.blogs.nytimes.com/2016/03/07/intermittent-fasting-diets-are-gaining-acceptance.
8. Thierry de Lestrade, *Le jeûne, une nouvelle thérapie?* (Paris: La Découverte, 2015), 35–55.
9. de Lestrade, *Le jeûne*, 79. In 2010, Thierry de Lestrade interviewed Dr. Nikolaev's son Valentin Nikolaev, who provided several quotations from his father.
10. de Lestrade, *Le jeûne*, 74.
11. de Lestrade, Le jeûne, 65–69.

12. Herbert Shelton, *The Science and Fine Arts of Fasting* (Mansfield Centre, CT: Martino, 2013), 464.
13. Arthur A. Daemmrich and Mary Ellen Bowden, "A Rising Drug Industry," *Chemical and Engineering News Archive* 83, no. 25 (2005): 28–42.
14. John Lear, "Taking the Miracle out of Miracle Drugs," *Saturday Review*, January 3, 1959, p. 35.
15. Lear, "Taking the Miracle out of Miracle Drugs," 39.
16. Sergey Ivanovich Filonov, *Dry Medical Fasting: Myths and Reality* (Barnaul, Siberia: Publishing House, 2008), 8.
17. Unless otherwise noted, all quotations and ideas attributed to Dr. Filonov come from my extensive interviews and conversations with him.

Chapter 17

1. Neil Nathan, *Toxic* (Las Vegas: Victory Belt, 2018), 8.
2. Nathan, *Toxic*, 39.
3. Suzanne Wu, "Fasting Triggers Stem Cell Regeneration of Damaged, Old Immune System," *USC News*, June 5, 2014, https://news.usc.edu/63669/fasting-triggers-stem-cell-regeneration-of-damaged-old-immune-system.
4. Anthony William, "Truth about Fasting," *Medical Medium Blog*, February 28, 2019, https://www.medicalmedium.com/blog/truth-about-fasting.
5. Sergey Ivanovich Filonov, *Dry Medical Fasting: Myths and Reality* (Barnaul, Siberia: Publishing House, 2008), 115.
6. Filonov, *Dry Medical Fasting*, 127.
7. Dale Bredeson, *The End of Alzheimer's: The First Program to Prevent and Reverse Cognitive Decline* (New York: Random House, 2017), 147.
8. National Institute on Aging, "International Symposium to Honor Pioneer in Neuroscience and Fasting," May 29, 2019, https://www.nia.nih.gov/news/international-symposium-honor-pioneer-neuroscience-and-fasting.

Chapter 18

1. Sergey Ivanovich Filonov, *Dry Medical Fasting: Myths and Reality* (Barnaul, Siberia: Publishing House, 2008), 7.
2. Rumi, *A Year with Rumi*, ed. Coleman Barks (New York: Harper Collins, 2006), 146.
3. Virginia Woolf, *On Being Ill* (Ashfield, MA: Paris Press, 2012), 12.
4. Herbert Shelton, *The Science and Fine Arts of Fasting* (Mansfield Centre, CT: Martino, 2013), 28.
5. Mark P. Mattson, "What Doesn't Kill You . . . ," *Scientific American* 313, no. 1 (2015): 40–45.
6. Filonov, *Dry Medical Fasting*, 100.
7. Wim Hof Method, "Cold Therapy," accessed February 15, 2022, https://www.wimhofmethod.com/cold-therapy.
8. For more about the Personalized Nutrition Project, visit the project's website, at http://personalnutrition.org/AboutGuests.aspx.
9. Rumi, *The Essential Rumi*, trans. Coleman Barks (New York: Harper Collins, 2004), 193.

Chapter 19

1. Michael Pollan, *In Defense of Food: An Eater's Manifesto* (New York: Penguin Press, 2008), 135.
2. Fred Bisci, *Your Healthy Journey* (New York: Bisci Lifestyle Books, 2009), 33.
3. Bisci, *Your Healthy Journey*, 33.
4. Danna Faulds, *Into the Heart of Yoga: One Woman's Journey* (Greenville, VA: Peaceable Kingdom Books, 2011), 331.

Epilogue

1. Danna Faulds, *Into the Heart of Yoga: One Woman's Journey* (Greenville, VA: Peaceable Kingdom Books, 2011), 22.
2. *The Upanishads*, trans. Eknath Easwaran (Tomales, CA: Blue Mountain Center of Meditation, 2007), 241.

BIBLIOGRAPHY

American Autoimmune Related Diseases Association. "Autoimmune Facts." Accessed February 15, 2022. https://autoimmune.org/wp-content/uploads/2019/12/1-in-5-Brochure.pdf.

Baudelaire, Charles. *Œuvres complètes*. Edited by Claude Pichois and Jean Ziegler. Paris: Gallimard, 1976.

Bazalgette, Louise, William Bradley, and Jenny Ousbey. *The Truth about Suicide*. London: Demos, 2011.

Berry, Wendell. *The Mad Farmer Poems*. Berkeley, CA: Counterpoint, 2013.

Bisci, Fred. *Your Healthy Journey*. New York: Bisci Lifestyle Books, 2009.

Bransfield, Robert C. "Suicide and Lyme and Associated Diseases." *Neuropsychotic Disease and Treatment* 13 (2017): 1575–1587.

Bredeson, Dale. *The End of Alzheimer's*. New York: Random House, 2017.

Carson, Rachel. *Silent Spring*. New York: Houghton Mifflin, 2002.

Centers for Disease Control and Prevention. "How Many People Get Lyme Disease?" January 13, 2021. https://www.cdc.gov/lyme/stats/humancases.html.

———."Lyme Disease." October 1, 2020. https://www.cdc.gov/ticks/tickbornediseases/lyme.html.

Cummings, E. E. "i thank You God for most this amazing." In *Complete Poems, 1904–1962*. Edited by George James Firmage. New York: Liveright, 2008.

Daemmrich, Arthur A., and Mary Ellen Bowden. "A Rising Drug Industry." *Chemical and Engineering News Archive* 83, no. 25 (2005): 28–42.

de Lestrade, Thierry. *Le jeûne, une nouvelle thérapie*. Paris: La Découverte, 2013.

Dewey, Edward. *The True Science of Living*. London: Henry Bill, 1895.

Duan, Lihua, Xiaoquan Rao, and Keshav Raj Sigdel. "Regulation of Inflammation in Autoimmune Disease." *Journal of Immunology Research*, February 28, 2019. https://doi.org/10.1155/2019/7403796.

Faulds, Danna. *Go In and In: Poems from the Heart of Yoga*. Greenville, VA: Morris Press, 2002.

———. *Into the Heart of Yoga: One Woman's Journey*. Greenville, VA: Peaceable Kingdom Books, 2011.

Filonov, Sergey. *Dry Fasting: 20 Questions and Answers*. Moscow: Siberika, 2019.

———. *Dry Medical Fasting: Myths and Reality*. Barnaul, Siberia: Publishing House, 2008.

Halperin, John J. "Neurologic Manifestations of Lyme Disease." *Current Infectious Disease Reports* 13, no. 4 (2011): 360–366.

Hinckley, Alison F., Neeta P. Connally, James I. Meek, Barbara J. Johnson, Melissa M. Kemperman, Katherine A. Feldman, Jennifer L. White, and Paul S. Mead. "Lyme Disease Testing by Large Commercial Laboratories in the United States." *Clinical Infectious Diseases* 59, no. 5 (2014): 676–681.

Johns Hopkins Bloomberg School of Public Health. "Lyme Disease Costs Up to $1.3 Billion per Year, Study Finds." February 5, 2015. https://publichealth.jhu.edu/2015/lyme-disease-costs-more-than-one-billion-dollars-per-year-to-treat-study-finds.

Jurgenson, Aivar. "The Formation of Siberian Identity and One of Its Political Manifestations." *Acta Historica Tallinnensia* 11 (2007): 30–47.

Kolata, Gina, and Sewell Chan. "Yoshinori Ohsumi of Japan Wins Nobel Prize for Study of 'Self-Eating' Cells." *New York Times*, October 3, 2016. https://www.nytimes.com/2016/10/04/science/yoshinori-ohsumi-nobel-prize-medicine.html.

Lear, John. "Taking the Miracle out of Miracle Drugs." *Saturday Review*, January 3, 1959, pp. 35–41.

London, Jack. *The Call of the Wild*. New York: Macmillan, 1919.

Longo, Valter. *The Longevity Diet*. New York: Random House, 2018.

Mattson, Mark P. "What Doesn't Kill You . . ." *Scientific American* 313, no. 1 (2015): 40–45.

———. "Why Fasting Bolsters Brain Power." TEDx Talks, March 18, 2014. https://www.youtube.com/watch?v=4UkZAwKoCP8.

Murphy, Dervla. *Full Tilt: Ireland to India with a Bicycle*. London: Eland, 2010.

Nathan, Neil. *Toxic*. Las Vegas: Victory Belt, 2018.

National Institute on Aging. "International Symposium to Honor Pioneer in Neuroscience and Fasting." May 29, 2019. https://www.nia.nih.gov/news/international-symposium-honor-pioneer-neuroscience-and-fasting.

National Institutes of Health. "Progress in Autoimmune Diseases Research." March 2005. https://www.niaid.nih.gov/sites/default/files/adccfinal.pdf.

Nikhilananda and Śaṅkarācārya. *The Upanishads*. New York: Harper, 1953.

O'Connor, Anahad. "Fasting Diets Are Gaining Acceptance." *New York Times*, March 7, 2016. https://well.blogs.nytimes.com/2016/03/07/intermittent-fasting-diets-are-gaining-acceptance.

Ogden, Nicholas H., Milka Radojevic, Xiaotian Wu, Venkata R. Duvvuri, Patrick A. Leighton, and Jianhong Wu. "Estimated Effects of Projected Climate Change on the Basic Reproductive Number of the Lyme Disease Vector Ixodes Scapularis." *Environmental Health Perspectives* 122, no. 6 (2014): 631–638.

Ohsumi, Yoshinori. Nobel Prize banquet speech. Stockholm, December 10, 2016. Available at https://www.nobelprize.org/prizes/medicine/2016/ohsumi/speech.

O'Rourke, Meghan. *Sun in Days: Poems*. New York: W. W. Norton, 2017.

Patanjali. *Yoga Sutras of Patanjali*. Calcutta: Susil Gupta, 1952.

Phillips, Steven, and Dana Parish. *Chronic: The Hidden Cause of the Autoimmune Pandemic and How to Get Healthy Again*. New York: Houghton Mifflin Harcourt, 2020.

Pollan, Michael. *In Defense of Food: An Eater's Manifesto*. New York: Penguin Press, 2008.

———. *The Omnivore's Dilemma: A Natural History of Four Meals*. New York: Penguin Press, 2006.

Pormann, Peter E. *The Cambridge Companion to Hippocrates*. Cambridge: Cambridge University Press, 2018.

Romm, Joseph. *Climate Change: What Everyone Needs to Know*. Oxford: Oxford University Press, 2015.

Rumi. *The Analects of Rumi*. Edited by Akṣapāda. N.p.: independently published, 2019.

———. *The Essential Rumi*. Translated by Coleman Barks. New York: Harper Collins, 2004.

———. *The Rumi Collection*. Edited by Kabir Helminski. London: Shambhala, 2012.

———. *A Year with Rumi*. Edited by Coleman Barks. New York: Harper Collins, 2006.

Shelton, Herbert. *Fasting Can Save Your Life*. Tampa: American Natural Hygiene Society, 1978.

———. *The Science and Fine Arts of Fasting*. Mansfield Centre, CT: Martino, 2013.

Sinclair, Upton. *The Fasting Cure*. New York: M. Kennerley, 1911.

Stranahan, Alexis, and Mark Mattson. "Recruiting Adaptive Cellular Stress Responses for Successful Brain Ageing." *Nature* 492, no. 7427 (2012): 209–216.

Tan, Amy. *The Opposite of Fate: A Book of Musings*. New York: G. P. Putnam's Sons, 2003.

The Upanishads. Translated by Eknath Easwaran. Tomales, CA: Blue Mountain Center of Meditation, 2007.

van der Kolk, Bessel. *The Body Keeps the Score: Brain, Mind, and Body in the Healing of Trauma*. New York: Penguin Books, 2014.

Versini, Mathilde, Pierre-Yves Jeandel, Eric Rosenthal, and Yehuda Shoenfeld. "Obesity in Autoimmune Diseases: Not a Passive Bystander." *Autoimmunity Reviews* 13, no. 9 (2014): 981–1000.

Whitman, Walt. *Leaves of Grass*. New York: Penguin Books, 2005.

William, Anthony. “Truth about Fasting.” *Medical Medium Blog*, February 28, 2019. https://www.medicalmedium.com/blog/truth-about-fasting.

Wim Hof Method. “Cold Therapy.” Accessed February 15, 2022. https://www.wimhofmethod.com/cold-therapy.

Wittgenstein, Ludwig. *Philosophical Investigations*. Translated by G. E. M. Anscombe. Oxford: Blackwell, 2001.

Woolf, Virginia. *On Being Ill*. Middletown, CT: Paris Press, 2012.

Wu, Suzanne. “Fasting Triggers Stem Cell Regeneration of Damaged, Old Immune System.” *USC News*, June 5, 2014. https://news.usc.edu/63669/fasting-triggers-stem-cell-regeneration-of-damaged-old-immune-system.

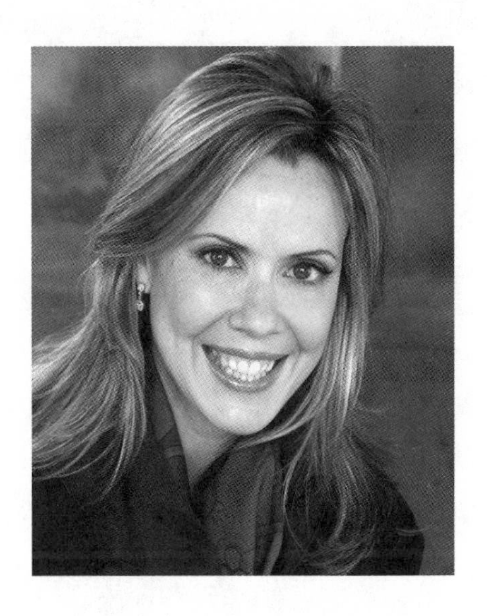

ABOUT THE AUTHOR

MICHELLE SLATER is a scholar of comparative literature and president of the educational nonprofit Mayapple Center for the Arts and Humanities in Connecticut. She holds a Ph.D. in French literature from Johns Hopkins University.

Her long battle with and recovery from late-stage neurological Lyme disease served as the genesis for this book. Debilitated by the disease to the extent that she was no longer able to teach at her university or perform simple tasks she used to take for granted, Slater spent several years pursuing every known treatment, from aggressive allopathic methods to holistic remedies. When all failed to deliver recovery, she discovered Dr. Sergey Filonov's dry-fasting program and spent two months in Siberia under his care. She recovered completely from Lyme disease, regaining her memory and returning to researching, writing books, hiking, and running. Since 2017, she has not experienced a single symptom.